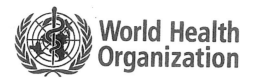

World Health Organization

CORRIGENDUM

Pandemic Influenza Preparedness and Response

ISBN 978 92 4 154768 0

- Page 32, reference 31 - Resolution WHA 58.5 Prevention and Control of influenza pandemics and annual epidemics - change to Strengthening pandemic influenza preparedness and response

- Page 32, reference 32 - Resolution WHA 58.5 Strengthening pandemic influenza preparedness and response

- Page 33, references 34 and 37 Resolution WHA 58.5 Strengthening pandemic influenza preparedness and response

D0898945

**GLOBAL
INFLUENZA
PROGRAMME**

PANDEMIC INFLUENZA
PREPAREDNESS AND
RESPONSE

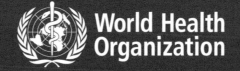
World Health
Organization

This guidance is an update of WHO Global Influenza Preparedness Plan, The role of *WHO and recommendations for national measures before and during pandemics*, published by WHO March 2005.[1]

FOREWORD

These guidelines were edited by Keiji Fukuda, Hande Harmanci, Kidong Park, Mary Chamberland, Elisabeth (*Isis*) Pluut, Tamara Curtin Niemi, Claudia Vivas and Jum Kanokporn Coninx of the Global Influenza Programme in the Health Security and Environment Cluster of the World Health Organization.

This guidance is an update of *WHO Global Influenza Preparedness Plan, The role of WHO and recommendations for national measures before and during pandemics,* published by WHO March 2005.[1]

The information and recommendations contained in this guidance is the product of expert opinion, derived from several international consultations which included examination of available information and modeling studies, input from public health experts on lessons learned from SARS and both animal and human influenza responses, and consolidation of recommendations in existing WHO guidance. This guidance was subject to an extensive public review. All external experts and contributors for all meetings and consultations, including those in the public review, have signed a declaration of interest statement in accordance with WHO policy. A small number of participants indicated a conflict of interest. However it was deemed by the working group that these declarations were not sufficient in conflict with the recommendations, to exclude them from the guidance development process. The declarations of interest are available upon request. For more information on the revision process, see Annex 2.

The Global Influenza Programme will revise this guidance in 2014, or sooner in the event of significant developments which impact pandemic preparedness and response planning.

1. WHO Global Influenza Preparedness Plan. The role of WHO and recommendations for national measures before and during pandemics, World Health Organization. 2005 (WHO/CDS/CSR/GIP/2005.5)

ACKNOWLEDGEMENTS

WHO wishes to acknowledge the contributions of experts from all over the world who participated in the process of developing this guidance:

P Abi-Hanna (Lebanon), L Ahadzie (Ghana), S Al Awaidy (Oman), T Asikainen (ECDC), Azimal (Indonesia), N Bakirci (Turkey), D Bell (USA), Y Berhane (Ethiopia), M Betancourt-Cravioto (Mexico), F Binam (Cameroon), D Boakye (Ghana), M Bökkerink (Netherlands), S Borroto-Gutierrez (Cuba), H Branswell (Canada), JS Bresee (USA), P Calvi-Parisetti (IFRC), D Camus (France), O Carlino (Argentina), E Carmo (Brazil), M de Carvalho (Brazil), M Cetron (USA), P Chappe (France), É Chatigny (Canada), P-H Chung (China), S Chunsuttiwat (Thailand), E Coker (Nigeria), T Colgate (IFPMA), J Cutter (Singapore), J Dabanch (Chile), V Davidyants (Armenia), B Duncan (ECDC), P Duplessis (IFRC), R El-Aouad (Morroco), O Ergonul (Turkey), B Eshaya-Chauvin (IFRC), M Esveld (Netherlands), R Fasce (Chile), M Fawzi (Egypt), N Fergusson (UK), L Finelli (USA), A Fiore (USA), G Foliot (WFP), A Fry (USA), J Gale (Singapore), M Gastellu-Etchegorry (France), N Gay (UK), U Go (Republic of Korea), P Grove (UK), MM Gouya (Iran), W Haas (Germany), J Hall (Australia), N Hehme (IFPMA), M Henkens (Belgium), N-T Hien (Vietnam), P Hung (Vietnam), P Imnadze (Georgia), M Jacobs (New Zealand), S Jadhav (DCVMN), A Kandeel (Egypt), M Kaku (Japan), G Kamenov (Bulgaria), F Karcher (EC), R Kirby (UK), O Kiselev (Russia), P Kreidl (ECDC), J-W Kwon (Republic of Korea), H-S Lee (Republic of Korea), W Lum (Panama), J Macey (Canada), J Mackenzie (Australia), H Mambu-ma-Disu (Congo), O Mansoor (UNICEF), M Mapatano (DR Congo), A Marx (OCHA), M Meltzer (USA), Z Memish (Saudi Arabia), Z Mohamed (Sudan), A Monto (USA), J Moran (Kazakhstan), M Mosselmans (OCHA), A Mounts (USA), Y Ndao (Senegal), H Needham (ECDC), J Newstead (UK), J Nguyen van Tam (UK), A Nicoll (ECDC), T Omori (Japan), H Oshitani (Japan), J O'Toole (ECDC), J Paget (Netherlands), E Palacios-Zavala (Mexico), B Paton (OCHA), C Patterson (Australia), W Peerapatanapokin (Thailand), E Perez (France), N Phin (UK), S Plotkin (USA), N Pshenichnaya (Russia), G Ramirez-Prada (Peru), P Ravindran (India), B Rawal (IFPMA), S Redd (USA), A Reynolds (UK), A Ricol-Solernou (EC), B Rodriques (UNICEF), C Russell (UK), G Saour (France), C Schuyler (NATO), J Sciberras (Canada), P Scott-Bowden (WFP), P Seukap (Cameroon), H Shirley-Quirk (UK), Y Shu (China), L Simonssen (USA), M Smolinski (USA), R Snacken (Belgium), S Strickland (UK), N Sunderland (USA), K Taniguchi (Japan), M Tashiro (Japan), J Toessi (Benin), B Toussaint (EC), P Tull (Sweden), M Vanderford (USA), M Van der Sande (Netherlands), S Vaux (France), L Vedrasco (OCHA), S Venkatesh (India), R Vivarie (UNHCR), S Vong (Cambodia), R Waldman (USA), W Wang (China), J Watson (UK), D Xiao (China), P Yosephine (Indonesia), H Yu (China), S Zaidi (Pakistan), H Zhao (UK), D Zoutman (Canada).

The following WHO staff were involved in the development and review of this document and their contribution is gratefully acknowledged:

B Abela-Ridder, W Alemu, C Alfonso, M Almiron, R Andraghetti, P Andrea, N Asgari, J Azé, M Barbeschi, P Ben-Embarek, I Bott, B Brennan, S Briand, C Brown, R Brown, P Carrasco, L Castellanos, M Chamberland, C Chauvin, M Chu, S Chungong, M Coly, P Cox, A Croisier, T Curtin-Niemi, A Dabbagh, T dos Santos, H El Bushra, N Eltantawys, N Emiroglu, S Eremin, D Featherstone, J Fitzner, M Friede, K Fukuda, B Ganter, M Gayer, P Ghimire, A Gilsdorf, T Grein, M Guardo, P Gully, M Hardiman, H Harmanci, G Hartl, F Hayden, M Hegermann-Lindencrone, D Heymann, H Hollmeyer, A Huvos, J Kanokporn Coninx, T Kasai, S Kirori, D Lavanchy, R Lee, D Legros, A Li, K Limpakarnjanarat, J Lopez-Macedo, Q Lui, C Maher, S Martin, D Menucci, A Merianos, C Mukoya, L Mumford, A Odugleh-Kolev, K O'Neill, S Otsu, L Palkonyay, K Park, C Pessoa Da Silva, O Pinheiro de Oliva, B Plotkin, S Pooransingh, G Poumerol, E Pluut, K Prosenc, J Rainford, A Reis, G Rodier, J Rovira, M Ryan, D Scales, N Shindo, C Toscano, K Vandemaele, C Vivas, J Watson, S Westman, E Whelan, S Wilburn, L Wolfson, A Yada, A Yeneabat, W Zhang, W Zhou, P Zuber

CONTENTS

FOREWORD   03

ACKNOWLEDGEMENTS   04

EXECUTIVE SUMMARY   08

1. INTRODUCTION   12

2. BACKGROUND   13
  2.1 **How influenza viruses with pandemic potential develop**   14
  2.2 **Ensuring ethical pandemic preparedness and response**   15
  2.3 **Integrating pandemic preparedness and response into general emergency preparedness**   15

3. ROLES AND RESPONSIBILITIES IN PREPAREDNESS AND RESPONSE   16
  3.1 **National preparedness and response as a whole-of-society responsibility**   16
    3.1.1 Government Leadership   17
    3.1.2 Health sector   17
    3.1.3 Non-health sectors   17
    3.1.4 Communities, individuals, and families 18
  3.2 **WHO**   18
    3.2.1 Coordination under International Health Regulations (IHR 2005)   19
    3.2.2 The designation of the global pandemic phase   20
    3.2.3. Switching to pandemic vaccine production   20
    3.2.4 Rapid containment of the initial emergence of pandemic influenza   21
    3.2.5 Providing an early assessment of pandemic severity on health   22

4. THE WHO PANDEMIC PHASES   24
  4.1 **Definition of the phases**   25
  4.2 **Phase changes**   26

5. RECOMMENDED ACTIONS BEFORE, DURING AND AFTER A PANDEMIC   28
  A. **Phases 1-3**   31
  B. **Phase 4**   36
  C. **Phases 5-6**   41
  D. **The post-peak period**   45
  E. **The post-pandemic period**   48

ANNEX 1 - PLANNING ASSUMPTIONS 49

1. Modes of transmission 49
    Suggested assumptions 49
    Implications 49
    Scientific basis 50
    Selected References 50

2. Incubation period and infectiousness of pandemic influenza 50
    Suggested assumptions 50
    Implications 51
    Scientific basis 51
    Selected References 51

3. Symptom development and clinical attack rate 52
    Suggested assumptions 52
    Implications 52
    Scientific basis 52
    Selected References 53

4. Dynamics of the pandemic and its impact 54
    Suggested assumptions 54
    Implications 54
    Scientific basis 54
    Selected References 55

ANNEX 2 REVISION PROCESS 56

EXECUTIVE SUMMARY

Influenza pandemics are unpredictable but recurring events that can have severe consequences on human health and economic well being worldwide. Advance planning and preparedness are critical to help mitigate the impact of a global pandemic. This WHO guidance document *Pandemic influenza preparedness and response* significantly updates and replaces *WHO global influenza preparedness plan: The role of WHO and recommendations for national measures before and during pandemics* which was published in 2005.

Why update the 2005 Guidance?

The global response to the spread of avian influenza A (H5N1) that began in 2003 has helped shape a number of significant public health advances. First, avian and pandemic influenza initiatives have led to substantial gains in strengthening national and global capacities and building partnerships between animal and human health sectors. Extensive practical experience in dealing with outbreaks of avian influenza (H5N1) virus in poultry and humans in addition to pandemic preparedness and response exercises carried out in various countries, has led to a greater understanding of the issues that need to be addressed in pandemic preparedness. Second, there is increased understanding of past pandemics, strengthened outbreak communications, greater insight into disease spread and approaches to control, and development of increasingly sophisticated statistical modeling techniques. Third, there has been growing attention to global health security following the adoption of revised International Health Regulations (IHR) in 2005 which provide a framework to address international public health concerns. Finally, stockpiles of antiviral drugs and other essential supplies are now a reality, new approaches to influenza vaccine development are under way and a Global Vaccine Action Plan[2] has been devised to increase the supply of pandemic vaccine.

Overview of the major changes

The revised Guidance:

1. **Retains the six-phase structure but regroups and redefines the phases to more accurately reflect pandemic risk and the epidemiological situation based upon observable phenomena.**
2. **Highlights key principles when undertaking pandemic planning including:**
   a) Application of ethical principles to assist policymakers in balancing a range of interests and protecting human rights;
   b) Integration of pandemic preparedness and response into national emergency frameworks to encourage sustainable preparedness;
   c) Incorporation of a "whole of society" approach that emphasizes not only the central role played by the health sector, but also the significant roles of other sectors such as businesses, families, communities and individuals.
3. **Harmonizes the recommended measures with the IHR 2005 and the concurrent development/revision of WHO guidance in related areas such as pandemic influenza surveillance, disease control measures, rapid containment and communications.**
4. **Includes suggested planning assumptions, their implications and a selected evidence base to aide planning efforts on a national level.**

---

2. Global pandemic influenza action plan to increase vaccine supply (WHO/CDS/EPR/GIP/2006.1) World Health Organization, 2006. (http://www.who.int/csr/resources/publications/influenza/WHO_CDS_EPR_GIP_2006_1/en/index.html, accessed 23 March 2009).

How to use this Guidance

This document should be used as a guide to inform and harmonize national and international preparedness and response before, during and after an influenza pandemic. Countries should develop or update national influenza preparedness and response plans that address the recommendations in this Guidance. This document is not intended to replace national plans which should be developed by each country.

This Guidance serves as the core strategic document in a suite of materials. It is supported by a complement of pandemic preparedness materials and tools (Figure 1). These documents and tools provide detailed information on a broad range of specific recommendations and activities, as well as clear guidance on their implementation. The individual elements of the guidance package will be made available as they are finalized.

FIGURE 1
THE WHO GUIDANCE PACKAGE FOR PANDEMIC INFLUENZA PREPAREDNESS AND RESPONSE

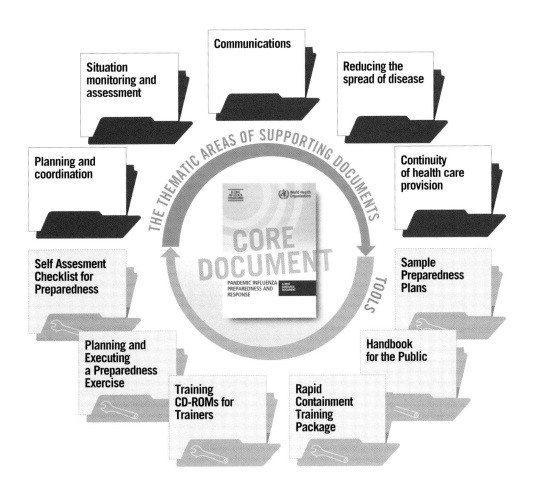

Roles and responsibilities in preparedness and response

A "whole-of-society" approach to pandemic influenza preparedness emphasizes the significant roles played by all sectors of society.

- The national government is the natural leader for communication and overall coordination efforts. Central governments should work to put in place the necessary legislation, policies and resources for pandemic preparedness, capacity development and anticipated response efforts across all sectors.
- The health sector (including public health and health care services) provides critical epidemiological, clinical and virological information which, in turn, informs measures to reduce spread of the pandemic virus and its attendant morbidity and mortality.
- The diverse array of non-health sectors must provide essential operations and services during a pandemic to mitigate health, economic and social impacts.
- Civil society organizations are often well placed to raise awareness, communicate accurate information, counter rumours, provide needed services, and liaise with the government during an emergency.
- Families and individuals can help reduce the spread of pandemic influenza through adoption of measures such as covering coughs and sneezes, hand washing, and the voluntary isolation of persons with respiratory illness.

WHO will work with Member States across a range of activities, including:

- Coordination of the international public health response under IHR 2005.
- Designation of the current global pandemic phase.
- Selection of the pandemic vaccine strain and recommendation of timing to start pandemic vaccine production.
- Assistance to national pandemic rapid containment efforts.
- Assessment of pandemic severity
- Global aggregation of key epidemiologic, virologic, and clinical information about the pandemic virus to help national authorities in deciding the optimal response.
- Provision of guidance and technical assistance.

The WHO pandemic phases

The phases are applicable globally and provide a framework to aid countries in pandemic preparedness and response planning. The use of a six-phased approach has been retained to facilitate incorporation of new recommendations into existing national plans. However, the pandemic phases have been re-defined (Table 1). To facilitate planning at national and global levels, Phases 1-3 and 5-6 have been grouped to include common action points. In addition, the time after the first pandemic wave has been elaborated into post peak and post pandemic periods. When making a change to the global phase, WHO will carefully consider all available information to assess if the criteria for a new phase have been met.

TABLE 1
PANDEMIC PHASE DESCRIPTIONS

	DESCRIPTION
PHASE 1	No animal influenza virus circulating among animals has been reported to cause infection in humans.
PHASE 2	An animal influenza virus circulating in domesticated or wild animals is known to have caused infection in humans and is therefore considered a specific potential pandemic threat.
PHASE 3	An animal or human-animal influenza reassortant virus has caused sporadic cases or small clusters of disease in people, but has not resulted in human-to-human transmission sufficient to sustain community-level outbreaks.
PHASE 4	Human-to-human transmission (H2H) of an animal or human-animal influenza reassortant virus able to sustain community-level outbreaks has been verified.
PHASE 5	The same identified virus has caused sustained community level outbreaks in two or more countries in one WHO region.
PHASE 6	In addition to the criteria defined in Phase 5, the same virus has caused sustained community level outbreaks in at least one other country in another WHO region.
POST-PEAK PERIOD	Levels of pandemic influenza in most countries with adequate surveillance have dropped below peak levels.
POSSIBLE NEW WAVE	Level of pandemic influenza activity in most countries with adequate surveillance rising again.
POST-PANDEMIC PERIOD	Levels of influenza activity have returned to the levels seen for seasonal influenza in most countries with adequate surveillance.

Recommended actions before, during and after a pandemic

Recommended actions to be taken by WHO and national authorities are presented for Phases 1-3, Phase 4, Phases 5-6, a post-peak period and a post-pandemic period. These actions are organized into the five basic components of preparedness and response:

1. **planning and coordination**
2. **situation monitoring and assessment**
3. **reducing the spread of disease**
4. **continuity of health care provision**
5. **communications**

Actions taken during Phases1-3 are aimed at strengthening pandemic preparedness and response capacities at global, regional, national and sub-national levels. The overarching goal of actions taken during Phase 4 is containment of the new virus within a limited area or the delay of its spread. If successful, valuable time could be gained to implement interventions including the use of vaccines. During Phases 5-6, actions shift from preparedness to response at a global level to reduce the impact of the pandemic. Actions during the post-peak period focus on addressing the health and social impact of the pandemic as well as preparation for a possible future pandemic wave(s). The focus of the post-pandemic period is restoration of normal health and social functions while addressing the long-term health and social impact of the pandemic.

Effectively meeting the challenges of the next influenza pandemic will require robust and extraordinary advance planning on the part of WHO and countries worldwide. WHO encourages countries to use this Guidance and the associated tools and supporting documents to build and strengthen national plans for pandemic influenza preparedness and response.

There is greater understanding that pandemic preparedness requires the involvement of not only the health sector, but the whole of society.

1. INTRODUCTION

WHO previously published pandemic preparedness guidance in 1999 and a revision of that guidance in 2005. Since 2005, there have been advances in many areas of preparedness and response planning. For example, stockpiles of antiviral drugs are now a reality and a WHO guideline[3] has been developed to attempt to stop or delay pandemic influenza at its initial emergence. There is increased understanding of past pandemics, strengthened outbreak communications, greater insight on disease spread and approaches to control, and increasingly sophisticated statistical modeling of various aspects of influenza. Extensive practical experience has been gained from responding to outbreaks of highly pathogenic avian influenza A (H5N1) virus infection in poultry and humans, and from conducting pandemic preparedness and response exercises in many countries. There is greater understanding that pandemic preparedness requires the involvement of not only the health sector, but the whole of society. In 2007, the International Health Regulations (2005) or IHR(2005) entered into force providing the international community with a framework to address international public health concerns.

In light of these developments, WHO decided to update its guidance to enable countries to be better prepared for the next pandemic. This Guidance serves as the core strategic document in a suite of materials. It is supported by a complement of pandemic preparedness materials and tools (Figure 1). These documents and tools provide detailed information on a broad range of specific recommendations and activities, as well as clear guidance on their implementation. The individual elements of the guidance package will be made available as they are finalized.

---

3. *WHO Interim Protocol: Rapid operations to contain the initial emergence of pandemic influenza.* World Health Organization, (http://www.who.int/csr/disease/avian_influenza/guidelines/draftprotocol/en/index.html, accessed 10 February, 2009)

Developing and sustaining a country's preparedness is challenging, and carries a risk of complacency.

2. BACKGROUND

Influenza pandemics are unpredictable but recurring events that can have severe consequences on societies worldwide. Since the 16th century, influenza pandemics have been described at intervals ranging between 10 and 50 years[4] with varying severity and impact (TABLE 2).

TABLE 2 CHARACTERISTICS OF THE THREE PANDEMICS OF THE 20th CENTURY[5]							
PANDEMIC (DATE AND COMMON NAME)	AREA OF EMERGENCE	INFLUENZA A VIRUS SUBTYPE	ESTIMATED REPRODUCTIVE NUMBER	ESTIMATED CASE FATALITY RATE	ESTIMATED ATTRIBUTABLE EXCESS MORTALITY WORLDWIDE	AGE GROUPS MOST AFFECTED (SIMULATED ATTACK RATES)	GDP LOSS (PERCENTAGE CHANGE)[6,7]
1918-1919 "Spanish Flu"	Unclear	H1N1	1.5-1.8	2-3%	20-50 million	Young adults	-16.9 to 2.4
1957-1958 "Asian Flu"	Southern China	H2N2	1.5	<0.2%	1-4 million	Children	-3.5 to 0.4
1968-1969 "Hong Kong Flu"	Southern China	H3N2	1.3-1.6	<0.2%	1-4 million	All age groups	-0.4 to (-1.5)

The precise timing and impact of a future influenza pandemic remains unknown. Developing and sustaining a country's preparedness is challenging, and carries a risk of complacency.

Pandemic preparedness in most, if not all countries, remains incomplete - even though an influenza pandemic could occur at any time resulting in:

- Rapid spread of pandemic disease leaving little time to implement ad hoc mitigation measures;
- Medical facilities struggling to cope with a possible large surge in demand;
- Potentially serious shortages of personnel and products resulting in disruption of key infrastructure and services, and continuity of all sectors of business and government;
- Delayed and limited availability of pandemic influenza vaccines, antivirals and antibiotics, as well as common medical supplies for treatment of other illnesses;
- Negative impact on social and economic activities of communities which could last long after the end of the pandemic period;
- Intense scrutiny from the public, government agencies, and the media on the state of national preparedness; and
- A global emergency limiting the potential for international assistance.

4. Avian influenza: assessing the pandemic threat. Geneva, World Health Organization, 2005 (WHO/CDS/2005.29).
5. Adapted from European Centre for Disease Prevention and Control, Pandemics of the 20th Century (http://ecdc.europa.eu/Health_topics/Pandemic_Influenza/stats.aspx accessed 6 October 2008).
6. McKibbin WJ, Sidorenko AA. Global Macroeconomic Consequences of Pandemic Influenza. Lowy Institute for International Policy. Analysis paper. Feb 2006. (http://www.acerh.edu.au/publications/McKibbin_PandemicFlu%20Report_2006.pdf accessed January 7, 2009).
7. McKibbin WJ, Sidorenko AA. The global cost of an influenza pandemic. The Milken Institute Review. Third Quarter 2007. (http://www.acerh.edu.au/publications/McKibbin_MilkenInstRev_2007.pdf accessed January 7, 2009).

2.1 How influenza viruses with pandemic potential develop

Many animal influenza viruses naturally infect and circulate among a variety of avian and mammalian species. Most of these animal influenza viruses do not normally infect humans. However, on occasion, certain animal viruses do infect humans. Such infections have most often occurred as sporadic or isolated infections or sometimes resulted in small clusters of human infections.

An influenza pandemic occurs when an animal influenza virus to which most humans have no immunity acquires the ability to cause sustained chains of human-to-human transmission leading to community-wide outbreaks. Such a virus has the potential to spread worldwide, causing a pandemic.

The development of an influenza pandemic can be considered the result of the transformation of an animal influenza virus into a human influenza virus. At the genetic level, pandemic influenza viruses may arise through:

- **Genetic reassortment:** a process in which genes from animal and human influenza viruses mix together to create a human-animal influenza reassortant virus;
- **Genetic mutation:** a process in which genes in an animal influenza virus change allowing the virus to infect humans and transmit easily among them.

2.1.1 The highly pathogenic avian influenza A (H5N1) virus and an influenza pandemic

In 1997, an avian influenza A virus of subtype H5N1 first demonstrated its capacity to infect humans after causing disease outbreaks in poultry in Hong Kong SAR, China. Since its widespread re-emergence in 2003-2004, this avian virus has resulted in millions of poultry infections and over four hundred human cases. An unusually high percentage of human H5N1 infections result in severe illness and death compared to other influenza viruses and far exceed the proportion of deaths caused by the 1918 pandemic virus. On rare occasions, H5N1 has spread from an infected person to another person - most often a family or other household member acting as a caregiver. However, none of these events has so far resulted in sustained community-level outbreaks.

The primary risk factor for a human to acquire a zoonotic H5N1 infection is direct contact or close exposure to infected poultry, although the virus remains difficult to transmit to humans. Five years after the widespread emergence and spread of H5N1, the virus is now entrenched in domestic birds in several countries. Controlling H5N1 among poultry is essential in reducing the risk of human infection and in preventing or reducing the severe economic burden of such outbreaks. Given the persistence of the H5N1 virus, successfully meeting this challenge will require long-term commitment from countries and strong coordination between animal and human health authorities.

While the H5N1 virus is currently the most visible influenza virus with pandemic potential, it is not the only candidate. Wild birds form a reservoir for a large number of other influenza viruses and influenza viruses are found in other animal species as well. Any one of these other viruses, which normally do not infect people, could transform into a pandemic virus. In addition to H5N1, other examples of animal influenza viruses previously known to infect people include avian H7 and H9 subtypes and swine influenza viruses. The H2 subtype, which was responsible for the 1957 pandemic (but has not circulated for decades), could also have the potential to cause a pandemic should it return. The uncertainty of the next pandemic virus means that planning for pandemic influenza should not exclusively focus on H5N1, but should be based on active and robust surveillance and science-based risk assessment.

2.2 Ensuring ethical pandemic preparedness and response

An influenza pandemic, like any urgent public health situation, calls for making certain decisions that will require balancing potentially conflicting individual interests with community interests. Policymakers can draw on ethical principles as tools to assess and balance these competing interests and values. An ethical approach does not provide a prescribed set of policies. Instead, it applies principles such as equity, utility /efficiency, liberty, reciprocity, and solidarity in light of local context and cultural values. While application of these principles sometimes results in competing claims, policymakers can use these principles as a framework to assess and balance a range of interests and to ensure that overarching concerns (such as protecting human rights and the special needs of vulnerable and minority groups) are addressed in pandemic influenza planning and response. Any measures that limit individual rights and civil liberties must be necessary, reasonable, proportional, equitable, non-discriminatory, and not in violation of national and international laws.[8]

WHO has developed[9] detailed ethical considerations on priority setting, disease control measures, the role and obligations of health care workers, and a multilateral response to pandemic influenza.

2.3 Integrating pandemic preparedness and response into general emergency preparedness

Pandemic preparedness activities take place within the context of national and international priorities, competing activities, and limited resources. Given the fundamental uncertainties surrounding the timing of the next influenza pandemic, steps to ensure the long-term sustainability of pandemic preparedness are crucial and should involve:

- Integration of pandemic influenza preparedness into national emergency preparedness plans, frameworks, and activities;
- Use of pandemic preparedness activities to strengthen basic and emergency health related capacities (such as the primary health care system, respiratory disease surveillance, and laboratory diagnostic capacities);
- Use of preparedness activities to actively build communication channels between sectors and communities;
- Development or modification of business continuity plans specifically tailored to pandemic influenza; and
- Periodic reassessment and updating of current plans based on new developments and information gained from exercises.

Through the use of these and other approaches, governments, public health agencies, and others have an opportunity to strengthen preparedness for the next influenza pandemic while building the capacity to address a range of local, national, and international emergencies.

8. *25 Questions and Answers on Health and Human Rights. Health and Human Rights* Publication Series Issue No.1, July 2002. World Health Organization. ISBN 92 4 154569 0, p 18.
9. *Ethical considerations in developing a public health response to pandemic influenza* (WHO/CDS/EPR/GIP/2007.2), World Health Organization, 2007.

While all sectors of society are involved in pandemic preparedness and response, the national government is the natural leader for overall coordination and communication efforts.

3. ROLES AND RESPONSIBILITIES IN PREPAREDNESS AND RESPONSE

3.1 National preparedness and response as a whole-of-society responsibility

A whole of society approach to pandemic influenza preparedness emphasizes the significant roles played by not only the health sector, but also all other sectors, individuals, families, and communities, in mitigating the effects of a pandemic. Developing capacities for mitigating the effects of a pandemic, including robust contingency and business continuity plans is at the heart of preparing the whole of society for a pandemic. Activities such as capacity development, planning, coordination, and communication are cross-cutting and require action by all parties (FIGURE 2).

FIGURE 2
WHOLE OF SOCIETY APPROACH TO PANDEMIC PREPAREDNESS

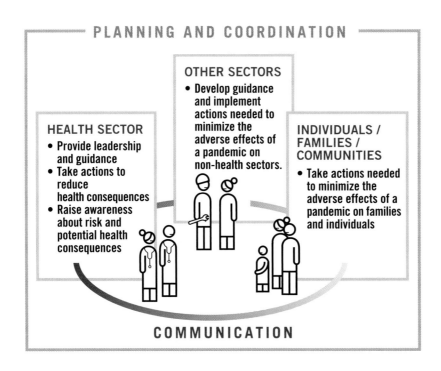

3.1.1 Government Leadership

While all sectors of society are involved in pandemic preparedness and response, the national government is the natural leader for overall coordination and communication efforts. In its leadership role, the central government should:

- Identify, appoint, and lead the coordinating body for pandemic preparedness and response; enact or modify legislation and policies required to sustain and optimize pandemic preparedness, capacity development, and response efforts across all sectors;
- Prioritize and guide the allocation and targeting of resources to achieve the goals as outlined in a country's Pandemic Influenza Preparedness Plan;
- Provide additional resources for national pandemic preparedness, capacity development, and response measures; and
- Consider providing resources and technical assistance to countries experiencing outbreaks of influenza with pandemic potential.

3.1.2 Health sector

The health sector (including public health and both public and private health care services), has a natural leadership and advocacy role in pandemic influenza preparedness and response efforts. In cooperation with other sectors and in support of national intersectoral leadership, the health sector must provide leadership and guidance on the actions needed, in addition to raising awareness of the risk and potential health consequences of an influenza pandemic. To fulfil this role, the health sector should be ready to:

- Provide reliable information on the risk, severity, and progression of a pandemic and the effectiveness of interventions used during a pandemic;
- Prioritize and continue the provision of health care during an influenza pandemic;
- Enact steps to reduce the spread of influenza in the community and in health care facilities; and
- Protect and support health care workers during a pandemic.

3.1.3 Non-health sectors

In the absence of early and effective preparedness, societies may experience social and economic disruption, threats to the continuity of essential services, reduced production, distribution difficulties, and shortages of essential commodities. Disruption of organizations may also have an impact on other businesses and services. For example, if electrical or water services are disrupted or fail, the health sector will be unable to maintain normal care. The failure of businesses would add significantly to the eventual economic consequences of a pandemic. Some business sectors will be especially vulnerable and certain groups in society are likely to suffer more than others. Developing robust preparedness and business continuity plans may enable essential operations to continue during a pandemic and significantly mitigate economic and social impacts. In order to minimize the adverse effects of a pandemic, all sectors should:

- Establish continuity policies to be implemented during a pandemic;
- Plan for the likely impact on businesses, essential services, educational institutions, and other organizations;
- Establish pandemic preparedness plans;

- Develop capacity and plan for pandemic response;
- Plan the allocation of resources to protect employees and customers;
- Communicate with and educate employees on how to protect themselves and on measures that will be implemented; and
- Contribute to cross-cutting planning and response efforts to support the continued functioning of the society.

3.1.4 Communities, individuals, and families

Civil society organizations, families, individuals, and traditional leaders all have essential roles to play in mitigating the effects of an influenza pandemic. Non-governmental groups should be involved in preparedness efforts and their expertise and capabilities harnessed to help communities prepare for and respond to a pandemic. The supporting document 'Whole-of-Society Pandemic Readiness' explores the roles of each of these groups in greater detail.[10]

Civil society organizations

Groups that have a close and direct relationship with communities are often well placed to raise awareness, communicate accurate information, counter rumours, provide needed services, and liaise with the government during an emergency. Such groups should identify their strengths and potential roles and, in partnership with local governments and other local organizations, plan for the actions they will take during a pandemic. These groups may be able to augment the efforts of organizations in other sectors, such as hospitals or clinics. For example, if large numbers of ill people are being cared for at home, community and faith-based organizations could provide support to households.

Individuals and families

During a pandemic, it is important that households take measures to ensure they have access to accurate information, food, water, and medicines. For families, access to reliable information from sources such as WHO and local and national governments will be essential. Individuals, especially those who have recovered from pandemic influenza, may consider volunteering with an organized group to assist others in the community.

Because influenza is transmitted from one person to another, the adoption of individual and household measures such as covering coughs and sneezes, hand washing, and the voluntary isolation of persons with respiratory illness may prevent additional infections.

3.2 WHO

WHO has been mandated by a series of World Health Assembly resolutions to provide Member States with guidance and technical support regarding influenza. These are listed below:

- **WHA 56.19:** Prevention and control of influenza pandemics and annual epidemics
- **WHA 58.5:** Strengthening pandemic influenza preparedness and response
- **WHA 60.28:** Pandemic influenza preparedness: Sharing of influenza viruses and access to vaccines and other benefits

---

10. *Whole of Society Pandemic Readiness*, World Health Organization 2009 (to be published 2009 to http://www.who.int/csr/disease/influenza/).

WHO will work with Member States across a range of activities, including coordination under the IHR (2005), designation of global pandemic phases, switching to pandemic vaccine production, coordination of a rapid containment operation, and providing early assessments of pandemic severity.

3.2.1 Coordination under International Health Regulations (IHR 2005)

The International Health Regulations (2005) also referred to as IHR (2005),[11] are an international legal instrument adopted by the World Health Assembly in 2005.[12] They are legally binding upon 194 States Parties around the world and provide a global legal framework to prevent, control, or respond to public health risks that may spread between countries.

Under the IHR (2005), a number of reporting requirements obligate States Parties to promptly inform WHO of cases or events involving a range of diseases and public health risks. These include the obligation to notify WHO of all cases of "human influenza caused by a new subtype" in their territories within 24 hours of assessment in accordance with the case definition established by WHO for this specific purpose.

These requirements, with related guidance on their application, are provided in Annex 2 of the IHR (2005). Notification must be followed by ongoing communication of detailed public health information on the event, including, where possible, case definitions, laboratory results, source and type of risk, number of cases and deaths, conditions affecting the spread of the disease, and the public health interventions employed. Even if there are no notifiable cases or events involving an influenza virus of pandemic potential occurring within a State, States Parties have additional obligations to report to WHO evidence of serious public health risks in other States, to the extent they have evidence of related imported or exported human cases. Finally, WHO has the mandate under the IHR (2005) to collect reports (including from unofficial sources) of potentially serious international public health risks and, after preliminarily assessment, to obtain verification of such reports from States.
If verification is sought, including in the context of potential pandemic influenza, States are required to respond to WHO within a prescribed time period and include available relevant public health information.[13,14]

All cases of human influenza of a new subtype, as further defined by WHO,
are notifiable to WHO under the IHR (2005).

In addition, all public health events, including those which may involve an influenza virus
of pandemic potential (even if not yet confirmed) are notifiable under the IHR (2005)
if they fulfil at least two of the contextual risk assessment criteria in the Regulations:

1.if the public health impact is serious;
2.if the event is unusual or unexpected;
3.if there is a significant risk of international spread; or
4.if there is a significant risk of international travel or trade restrictions.

11. World Health Organization. International Health Regulations (2005). ISBN 978 92 4 158041 0.
12. Resolution WHA 58.3 Revision of the International Health Regulations. In: Fifty-eighth World Health Assembly, Geneva 16-25 May, 2005 (WHA58/2005/REC/3).
13. World Health Organization. International Health Regulations (2005). ISBN 978 92 4 158041 0.
14. Plotkin, Hardiman, Gonzalez-Martin and Rodier, "Infectious disease surveillance and the International Health Regulations, Chapter 2 in Infectious Disease Surveillance. Blackwell Publishing 2007.

The IHR (2005) also obligates States Parties to develop national public health capacities to detect, assess and respond to events, and to report to WHO as necessary, as well as capacities to address risks of international spread of disease at designated ports and airports (and potentially, at designated ground crossings).[15] If a potential pandemic or related public health risk should arise, the IHR also provides extensive options for national authorities to obtain information from incoming aircraft, ships, and other vehicles and travellers, and includes the potential use of medical or public health interventions subject to various safeguards and other requirements. Regarding international travellers, for example, there are human rights and other protections, such as prior informed consent for examinations, prophylaxis or other measures (subject to exceptions in exigent circumstances). There are also obligations to provide adequate food, water, medical care, and other essentials to international travellers who are isolated or quarantined.[16]

The IHR (2005) also provides a mandate to WHO to perform public health surveillance, support States, and coordinate international response to international public health risks. In extraordinary circumstances, including an influenza pandemic, the Regulations provide that the WHO Director-General can determine that a "public health emergency of international concern" is occurring. In such a case, the Director-General will, after taking advice from a committee of outside experts, determine and issue specific IHR "Temporary Recommendations" to governments on the appropriate actions to prevent or reduce the international spread and minimize unnecessary interference with international traffic and trade. Both the determination that a Public Health Emergency of International Concern (PHEIC) is occurring (which may also require outside expert advice) and the issuance of Temporary Recommendations are based upon specific procedures and criteria in the IHR (2005).[17]

3.2.2 The designation of the global pandemic phase

The designation of the global pandemic phase will be made by the Director-General of WHO. The designation of a phase will be made consistent with applicable provisions of the IHR (2005) and in consultation with other organizations, institutions, and affected Member States.

3.2.3. Switching to pandemic vaccine production

One of WHO's critical actions during an emerging pandemic will be selection of the pandemic vaccine strain and determining the time to begin production of a pandemic vaccine instead of a seasonal influenza vaccine.

WHO issues bi-annual recommendations on the composition of seasonal influenza vaccines and, in addition, has been reviewing vaccine candidate viruses for A (H5N1) and other influenza subtypes with pandemic potential since 2004. This process is undertaken in consultation with WHO Collaborating Centres (*CCs*)[18] for influenza, National Influenza Centres, WHO H5 Reference Laboratories, and key national regulatory reference laboratories based on surveillance conducted by the WHO Global Influenza Surveillance Network (*GISN*). The recommendations and availability of vaccine viruses are announced in a public meeting and simultaneously on the WHO website,[19] and are also communicated to influenza vaccine manufacturers via the International Federation of Pharmaceutical Manufacturers and Associations and the Developing Country Vaccine Manufacturers Network.

15. World Health Organization. International Health Regulations (2005). ISBN 978 92 4 158041 0. Articles 5.1, 13.1 and Annex 1.
16. World Health Organization. International Health Regulations (2005). ISBN 978 92 4 158041 0. Articles 23.32, 37-8 and Annexes 8-9.
17. World Health Organization. International Health Regulations (2005). ISBN 978 92 4 158041 0.Articles 12, 15, 17-18, 48-49.
18. WHO Collaborating Centres and Reference Laboratories involved in annual influenza vaccine composition recommendations (http://www.who.int/csr/disease/influenza/collabcentres/en/index.html accessed 10 February 2009).
19. Recommendations for influenza vaccines (http://www.who.int/csr/disease/influenza/vaccinerecommendations, accessed 3 December 2008).

As soon as there is credible evidence to suggest that an influenza virus with pandemic potential has acquired the ability to sustain human-to-human transmission, WHO will expedite the process of review, selection, development, and distribution of vaccine viruses for pandemic vaccine production, as well as vaccine potency testing reagents and preparations involving all stakeholders as necessary. The efficiency of this process depends on the timely sharing of viruses/clinical specimens with WHO via GISN/WHO CCs.

If the situation involves parallel determination of a PHEIC by the Director-General, then the decision to recommend a vaccine switch in production will be taken with due consideration to applicable requirements under the IHR (2005), including potentially, advice from an IHR Emergency Committee as appropriate. WHO will then announce its recommendations on whether and when to switch production to pandemic vaccine and the virus strain that should be used in the pandemic vaccine.

Given the possible rapid spread of the pandemic virus and the potential consequences of a pandemic, as well as the time needed for vaccine production, the process to decide whether to switch to pandemic vaccine will be started independently from the formal declaration of a pandemic phase change.

3.2.4 Rapid containment of the initial emergence of pandemic influenza

The intention of a pandemic influenza rapid containment operation is for national authorities, with the assistance of WHO and international partners to prevent or delay the widespread transmission of an influenza virus with pandemic potential as soon as possible following its initial detection. Rapid pandemic containment is an extraordinary public health action, which builds upon, but goes beyond, routine outbreak response and disease control measures.

The WHO pandemic rapid containment guidance,[20] which is periodically reviewed and updated, outlines what should be done, provides information on how to do it, and serves as the foundation for the development of more detailed operational plans. Rapid containment poses a number of planning, resource, and organizational challenges. The exercising of operational components of pandemic preparedness and response plans, including elements related to pandemic rapid containment operations is strongly encouraged.

If a rapid containment operation is being considered, national authorities and WHO will need to jointly and rapidly assess all the relevant technical, operational, and political factors to determine if:

- Compelling evidence is present to suggest that an influenza virus with pandemic potentia has gained the ability to transmit efficiently from human-to-human at a level that can sustain community - level outbreaks; and
- There are compelling reasons why a containment operation should not be attempted.

A recommendation whether to proceed will depend on expert assessment of the situation and related scientific and operational feasibility factors. A rapid containment operation would likely not be attempted if evidence suggests that the virus with pandemic potential has already spread too widely to make containment feasible or if it was considered not operationally possible to rapidly implement the necessary measures. Should a decision be made to proceed, WHO will provide ongoing advice and support to the affected country on management and technical aspects of the containment operation. WHO will also support the coordination and implementation of international responses,

20. WHO Interim planning guidance for rapid containment of the initial emergence of pandemic influenza.
(http://www.who.int/csr/disease/avian_influenza/guidelines/draftprotocol/en/index.html accessed 10 February 2009).

such as the deployment of international field teams, if requested; mobilizing and dispatching necessary resources (e.g. antivirals and other materials); and developing or refining guidance in consultation with the affected country and external experts. Ultimately the decision to launch a rapid containment operation rests with the national authority. The announcement of Phase 4 is not required for rapid pandemic containment efforts as the decision to mount an operation could be made before or after a phase change.

Launching a containment operation will require time to mobilize and deploy equipment, people, and supplies. Before a formal decision has been made to initiate rapid containment, the affected country and WHO may need to initiate response activities if available information is highly suggestive, but not yet definitive, that an influenza virus capable of causing a pandemic has emerged.

National authorities and WHO will need to be in continuous communication and maintain a flexible and agile approach to the developing situation.

3.2.5 Providing an early assessment of pandemic severity on health

As soon as possible, WHO will provide an assessment of pandemic severity to help governments determine the level of interventions required as part of their response. As outlined in section 1.1, past influenza pandemics have been associated with varying levels of illness and death. Although making an informed assessment of severity early in the course of a pandemic will be challenging, such an assessment will assist countries in:

- Deciding whether or not to implement mitigation measures that may be potentially disruptive;
- Prioritizing the use of antivirals, vaccines, and other medical interventions;
- Managing continuity of health care; and
- Communicating with the media and the public and answering queries.

Pandemic severity may be assessed in many ways. One fundamental distinction is an assessment based on direct health effects as opposed to one based upon societal and economic effects. While societal and economic effects may be highly variable from country to country and dependent upon multiple factors (including the effects of the media and the underlying state of preparedness), WHO plans to assess pandemic severity based primarily on observable effects on health.[21]

Available quantitative and qualitative data on health impacts will be used to estimate severity using the three-point scale of Mild-Intermediate-Severe. As more information becomes available,

WHO will update the severity assessment. Since national circumstances will vary in terms of disease activity and capacity to respond, caution should be exercised in directly linking severity assessment at a global level to actions at the national level.

It is likely that information will be limited early in the pandemic while the demand for information simultaneously escalates. If pandemic surveillance is to provide sufficient information and data to assess severity, countries need to review their existing surveillance capacity to address the weaknesses to be prepared for pandemic surveillance. Essential components of an effective pandemic influenza surveillance system will include:

21. WHO Global Surveillance for Pandemic Influenza, World Health Organization 2009 (to be published 2009 http://www.who.int/csr/disease/influenza/).

- Early detection and investigation;
- Comprehensive assessment; and
- Monitoring.[22]

Potential health indicators of severity

- **Case fatality rate**
- **Unusually severe morbidity**
- **Unexpected mortality patterns**
- **Unusual complications**

22. WHO Global Surveillance for Pandemic Influenza, World Health Organization 2009 (to be published 2009 http://www.who.int/csr/disease/influenza/).

The grouping and description of pandemic phases have been revised to make them easier to understand, more precise, and based upon observable phenomena.

4. THE WHO PANDEMIC PHASES

The WHO pandemic phases were developed in 1999 and revised in 2005. The phases are applicable to the entire world and provide a global framework to aid countries in pandemic preparedness and response planning. In this revision, WHO has retained the use of a six-phased approach for easy incorporation of new recommendations and approaches into existing national preparedness and response plans. The grouping and description of pandemic phases have been revised to make them easier to understand, more precise, and based upon observable phenomena. Phases 1-3 correlate with preparedness, including capacity development and response planning activities, while Phases 4-6 clearly signal the need for response and mitigation efforts. Furthermore, periods after the first pandemic wave are elaborated to facilitate post pandemic recovery activities.

The 2009 pandemic phases are:
- a planning tool;
- simpler, more precise, and based on verifiable phenomena;
- will be declared in accordance with the IHR (2005);
- only loosely correspond to pandemic risk;
- identify sustained human-to-human transmission as a key event;
- better distinguish between time for preparedness and response; and
- include the post-peak and post-pandemic periods for recovery activities.

The new phases are **NOT**:
- designed to predict what will happen during a pandemic; and
- always going to proceed in numerical order.

FIGURE 3
PANDEMIC INFLUENZA PHASES (2009)

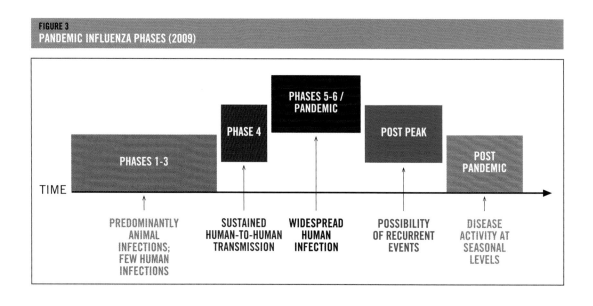

4.1 Definition of the phases

In nature, influenza viruses circulate continuously among animals, especially birds. Even though such viruses might theoretically develop into pandemic viruses, in **Phase 1** no viruses circulating among animals have been reported to cause infections in humans.

In **Phase 2** an animal influenza virus circulating among domesticated or wild animals is known to have caused infection in humans, and is therefore considered a potential pandemic threat.

In **Phase 3**, an animal or human-animal influenza reassortant virus has caused sporadic cases or small clusters of disease in people, but has not resulted in human-to-human transmission sufficient to sustain community-level outbreaks. Limited human-to-human transmission may occur under some circumstances, for example, when there is close contact between an infected person and an unprotected caregiver. However, limited transmission under such restricted circumstances does not indicate that the virus has gained the level of transmissibility among humans necessary to cause a pandemic.
Phase 4 is characterized by verified human-to-human transmission of an animal or human-animal influenza reassortant virus able to cause "community-level outbreaks." The ability to cause sustained disease outbreaks in a community marks a significant upwards shift in the risk for a pandemic. Any country that suspects or has verified such an event should urgently consult with WHO so that the situation can be jointly assessed and a decision made by the affected country if implementation of a rapid pandemic containment operation is warranted. Phase 4 indicates a significant increase in risk of a pandemic but does not necessarily mean that a pandemic is a forgone conclusion.

Phase 5 is characterized by human-to-human spread of the virus into at least two countries in one WHO region (Figure 5)[23]. While most countries will not be affected at this stage, the declaration of Phase 5 is a strong signal that a pandemic is imminent and that the time to finalize the organization, communication, and implementation of the planned mitigation measures is short.

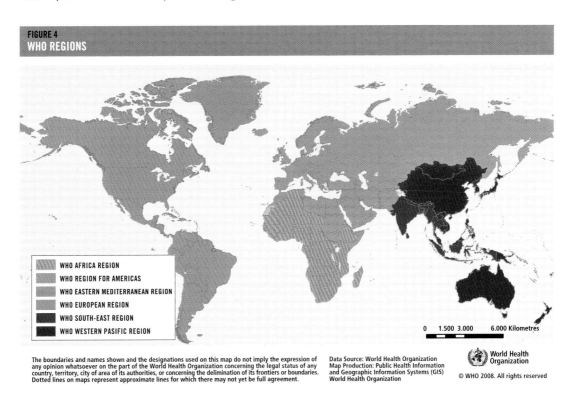

FIGURE 4
WHO REGIONS

WHO AFRICA REGION
WHO REGION FOR AMERICAS
WHO EASTERN MEDITERRANEAN REGION
WHO EUROPEAN REGION
WHO SOUTH-EAST REGION
WHO WESTERN PASIFIC REGION

0   1.500 3.000   6.000 Kilometres

The boundaries and names shown and the designations used on this map do not imply the expression of any opinion whatsoever on the part of the World Health Organization concerning the legal status of any country, territory, city of area of its authorities, or concerning the delimitation of its frontiers or boundaries. Dotted lines on maps represent approximate lines for which there may not yet be full agreement.

Data Source: World Health Organization
Map Production: Public Health Information and Geographic Information Systems (GIS)
World Health Organization

World Health Organization

© WHO 2008. All rights reserved

23. WHO - its people and offices (http://www.who.int/about/structure/en/index.html, accessed 10 February 2009).

Phase 6, the pandemic phase, is characterized by community level outbreaks in at least one other country in a different WHO region in addition to the criteria defined in **Phase 5**. Designation of this phase will indicate that a global pandemic is under way.

During the **post-peak** period, pandemic disease levels in most countries with adequate surveillance will have dropped below peak observed levels. The post-peak period signifies that pandemic activity appears to be decreasing; however, it is uncertain if additional waves will occur and countries will need to be prepared for a second wave.

Previous pandemics have been characterized by waves of activity spread over months. Once the level of disease activity drops, a critical communications task will be to balance this information with the possibility of another wave. Pandemic waves can be separated by months and an immediate "at-ease" signal may be premature.

In the **post-pandemic** period, influenza disease activity will have returned to levels normally seen for seasonal influenza. It is expected that the pandemic virus will behave as a seasonal influenza A virus. At this stage, it is important to maintain surveillance and update pandemic preparedness and response plans accordingly. An intensive phase of recovery and evaluation may be required.

This phased approach is intended to help countries and other stakeholders to anticipate when certain situations will require decisions and decide at which point main actions should be implemented (see TABLE 3). As in the 2005 guidance, each of the phases applies worldwide once announced. However, individual countries will be affected at different times. In addition to the globally announced pandemic phase, countries may want to make further national distinctions based upon their specific situations. For example, countries may wish to consider whether the potential pandemic virus is causing disease within their own borders, in neighbouring countries, or countries in close proximity.

4.2 Phase changes

It is important to stress that the phases were not developed as an epidemiological prediction, but to provide guidance to countries on the implementation of activities. While later phases may loosely correlate with increasing levels of pandemic risk, this risk in the first three phases is simply unknown. It is therefore possible to have situations which pose an increased pandemic risk, but do not result in a pandemic.

Alternatively, although global influenza surveillance and monitoring systems are much improved, it is also possible that the first outbreaks of a pandemic will not be detected or recognized. For example, if symptoms are mild and not very specific, an influenza virus with pandemic potential may attain relatively widespread circulation before being detected; thus, the global phase may jump from Phase 3 to Phases 5 or 6. If the rapid containment operations are successful, Phase 4 may revert back to Phase 3.

When making a change to the global phase, WHO will carefully consider whether the criteria for a new phase have been met. This decision will be based upon all credible information from global surveillance and from other organizations.[24]

---

24. Such as the Food and Agriculture Organization of the United Nations (FAO) and the World Organisation for Animal Health (OIE) for earlier phases.

TABLE 3
WHO PANDEMIC PHASE DESCRIPTIONS AND MAIN ACTIONS BY PHASE

	ESTIMATED PROBABILITY OF PANDEMIC	DESCRIPTION	MAIN ACTIONS IN AFFECTED COUNTRIES	MAIN ACTIONS IN NOT-YET-AFFECTED COUNTRIES
PHASE 1	Uncertain	No animal influenza virus circulating among animals has been reported to cause infection in humans.	Producing, implementing, exercising, and harmonizing national pandemic influenza preparedness and response plans with national emergency preparedness and response plans.	
PHASE 2		An animal influenza virus circulating in domesticated or wild animals is known to have caused infection in humans and is therefore considered a specific potential pandemic threat.		
PHASE 3		An animal or human-animal influenza reassortant virus has caused sporadic cases or small clusters of disease in people, but has not resulted in human-to-human transmission sufficient to sustain community-level outbreaks.		
PHASE 4	Medium to high	Human-to-human transmission of an animal or human-animal influenza reassortant virus able to sustain community-level outbreaks has been verified.	Rapid containment.	Readiness for pandemic response.
PHASE 5	High to certain	The same identified virus has caused sustained community level outbreaks in at least two countries in one WHO region.	Pandemic response: Each country to implement actions as called for in their national plans.	Readiness for imminent response.
PHASE 6	Pandemic in progress	In addition to the criteria defined in Phase 5, the same virus has caused sustained community level outbreaks in at least one other country in another WHO region.		
POST-PEAK PERIOD		Levels of pandemic influenza in most countries with adequate surveillance have dropped below peak levels.	Evaluation of response; recovery; preparation for possible second wave.	
POSSIBLE NEW WAVE		Level of pandemic influenza activity in most countries with adequate surveillance is rising again.	Response	-
POST-PANDEMIC PERIOD		Levels of influenza have returned to the levels seen for seasonal influenza in most countries with adequate surveillance.	Evaluation of response; revision of plans; recovery.	

The goal of planning and coordination efforts is to provide leadership and coordination across sectors.

5. RECOMMENDED ACTIONS BEFORE, DURING AND AFTER A PANDEMIC

This section provides specific actions to be taken by national authorities and WHO. The new WHO pandemic phases and a summary of recommended actions for each phase are presented in Table 4. Recommendations are grouped by pandemic phases and the five components of preparedness and response which are the following:

1. Planning and coordination
2. Situation monitoring and assessment
3. Reducing the spread of disease
4. Continuity of health care provision
5. Communications

The goal of **planning and coordination** efforts is to provide leadership and coordination across sectors. One important aspect is to integrate pandemic preparedness into national emergency preparedness frameworks.

The goal of **situation monitoring and assessment** is to collect, interpret, and disseminate information on the risk of a pandemic before it occurs and, once under way, to monitor pandemic activity and characteristics. To assess if the risk of a pandemic is increasing, it will be important to monitor the infectious agent, its capacity to cause disease in humans, and the patterns of disease spread in communities. It is important to collect data on influenza viruses, the genetic changes taking place and consequent changes in biological characteristics, and to rapidly investigate and evaluate outbreaks. Once a pandemic influenza virus begins to circulate, it will be vital to assess the effectiveness of the response measures.

Reducing the spread of disease will depend significantly upon increasing the "social distance" between people. Measures such as individual/household level measures, societal-level measures and international travel measures, and the use of antivirals, other pharmaceuticals, and vaccines will be important.

Individual/household level measures include risk communication, individual hygiene and personal protection, and home care of the ill and quarantine of contacts. *Societal-level measures* are applied to societies or communities rather than individuals or families. These measures require a behavioural change in the population, multiple sector involvement, mobilization of resources, strong communication, and media support.

International travel measures aim to delay the entry of pandemic disease into not-yet-affected countries and will have an impact on international traffic and trade. Countries should balance reducing the risks to public health and avoiding unnecessary interference with international traffic and trade.

The use of *pharmaceutical interventions* to prevent or treat influenza encompasses a range of approaches. Additionally, the successful prevention and treatment of secondary or pre-existing conditions will be a key factor in many settings for reducing the overall burden of illness and death.

During a pandemic, **health systems** will need to provide health care services while attending to the influx of patients with influenza illness. Planning for surge capacity in health care facilities will help determine the extent to which the existing health system can expand to manage the additional patient load. Health care facilities will need to maintain adequate triage and infection control measures to protect health care workers, patients, and visitors.

The goal of **communications** before and during a pandemic is to provide and exchange relevant information with the public, partners, and stakeholders to allow them to make well informed decisions and take appropriate actions to protect health and safety. Effective communication about the risks related to pandemic influenza is critical at every stage of preparedness and response and is a fundamental part of effective risk management. Communications should be based on the five principles outlined in WHO's Outbreak Communications Guide:[25] planning; trust; transparency; announcing early; and listening. Given the complex risks and perceptions associated with an influenza pandemic, communication strategies that simply disseminate outbreak information and recommendations will be insufficient. The scope and complexity of the task demands frequent, transparent, and proactive communication and information exchange with the public, partners, and other stakeholders about decision making, health recommendations, and related information. In addition to the suggested actions which follow below, countries are encouraged to develop core risk communication capacities such as those described in the WHO Outbreak Communication Planning Guide. By developing a solid foundation for pandemic influenza communications, Member States would also strengthen communication response systems for any public health emergency that may arise.

Core elements of pandemic influenza communication are:

- **to maintain and build public trust in public health authorities before, during and after an influenza pandemic;**
- **to support coordination and the efficient use of limited resources among local, national, regional and international public health partners;**
- **to provide relevant public health information to the public; to support vulnerable populations having the information they need to make well-informed decisions;**
- **to take appropriate actions to protect their health and safety; and**
- **to minimize social and economic disruption.**

25. World Health Organization Outbreak Communication Planning Guide. World Health Organization 2008. ISBN 978 92 4 159744 9.

TABLE 4
SUMMARY TABLE OF RECOMMENDED ACTIONS

PREPAREDNESS COMPONENTS	PHASES				
	1-3	4	5-6	POST PEAK	POST PANDEMIC
PLANNING AND COORDINATION	**Develop, exercise**, and periodically **revise** national influenza pandemic preparedness and response **plans.**	Direct and coordinate rapid pandemic **containment** activities in collaboration with WHO to limit or delay the spread of infection.	Provide **leadership** and **coordination** to **multisectoral resources** to mitigate the societal and economic impacts.	Plan and coordinate for **additional resources** and **capacities** during possible future waves.	**Review** lessons learned and share experiences with the international community. **Replenish** resources.
SITUATION MONITORING AND ASSESSMENT	**Develop** robust national **surveillance** systems in collaboration with national animal health authorities, and other relevant sectors.	**Increase** surveillance. Monitor containment operations. Share findings with WHO and the international community.	**Actively monitor and assess** the evolving pandemic and its impacts and mitigation measures.	**Continue** surveillance to detect subsequent waves.	**Evaluate** the pandemic characteristics and situation monitoring and assessment tools for the next pandemic and other public health emergencies.
COMMUNICATIONS	**Complete** communications planning and initiate **communications** activities to communicate real and potential risks.	Promote and communicate recommended **interventions** to prevent and reduce population and individual risk.	Continue **providing updates** to general public and all stakeholders on the state of pandemic and measures to mitigate risk.	**Regularly update** the public and other stakeholders on any changes to the status of the pandemic.	Publicly **acknowledge** contributions of all communities and sectors and communicate the lessons learned; **incorporate** lessons learned into communications activities and planning for the next major public health crisis.
REDUCING THE SPREAD OF DISEASE	**Promote beneficial behaviours** in individuals for self protection. Plan for use of pharmaceuticals and vaccines.	Implement rapid pandemic **containment** operations and other activities; collaborate with WHO and the international community as necessary.	**Implement** individual, societal, and pharmaceutical measures.	**Evaluate** the effectiveness of the measures used to update guidelines, protocols, and algorithms.	Conduct a **through evaluation** of all interventions implemented.
CONTINUITY OF HEALTH CARE PROVISION	**Prepare** the health system to **scale up.**	Activate **contingency** plans.	**Implement** contingency plans for health systems at all levels.	**Rest, restock** resources, **revise** plans, **and rebuild** essential services.	**Evaluate** the response of the health system to the pandemic *and* **share** *the lessons learned.*

PHASES 1-3

TABLE 5
ACTIONS FOR WHO AND NATIONAL AUTHORITIES, BY PHASE

A. PHASES 1-3

Actions taken during pandemic Phases 1-3 are aimed at strengthening pandemic influenza preparedness and response capacities at global, regional, national and sub-national levels.

26. Resolution WHA 56.19 Prevention and control of influenza pandemics and annual epidemics. In: Fifty-sixth World Health Assembly, Geneva 19-28 May, 2003
27. Resolution WHA 56.19 Prevention and control of influenza pandemics and annual epidemics. In: Fifty-sixth World Health Assembly, Geneva 19-28 May, 2003.
28. Resolution WHA 56.19 Prevention and control of influenza pandemics and annual epidemics. In: Fifty-sixth World Health Assembly, Geneva 19-28 May, 2003.
29. Ethical considerations in developing a public health response to pandemic influenza (WHO/CDS/EPR/GIP/2007.2), World Health Organization, 2007.

PHASES 1-3
PLANNING AND COORDINATION

WHO ACTIONS	NATIONAL ACTIONS
• Provide technical support to Member States in the preparation of national pandemic preparedness plans.[26]	• Establish and activate a cross-governmental, multi-agency national pandemic preparedness committee that meets regularly.
• Provide leadership in coordinating the prioritized activities for epidemic and pandemic preparedness.[27]	• Assess capacities and identify priorities for pandemic preparedness planning and response at national and sub-national levels.
• Advocate new partnerships with organizations of the United Nations system, bilateral development agencies, nongovernmental organizations, and the private sector.[28]	• Advise sub-national governments on best practices in pandemic planning; monitor and evaluate the operability and quality of their plans.
• Facilitate and encourage the operability of national pandemic plans through preparedness activities, including exercises.	• Develop, exercise, and periodically revise national and sub-national influenza pandemic preparedness and response plans in close collaboration with human and animal health sectors and other relevant public and private partners with reference to current WHO guidance.
	• Establish, as needed, full legal authority and legislation for all proposed interventions.
	• Anticipate and address the resources required to implement proposed interventions at national and sub-national levels including working with humanitarian, community-based, and non-governmental organizations.
	• Develop an ethical framework to govern pandemic policy development and implementation.[29]
	• Integrate pandemic preparedness and response plans into existing national emergency preparedness and response programmes.
	• Provide to public and private sectors the key assumptions, guidance and relevant information to facilitate their pandemic business continuity planning.
	• Identify and address trans-border issues, including interoperability of plans across borders.
	• Consider providing resources and technical assistance to resource-poor countries with foci of influenza activity.
	• Participate, when possible, in regional and international pandemic preparedness planning initiatives and exercises.

1-3 PREDOMINANTLY ANIMAL INFECTIONS; FEW HUMAN INFECTIONS

30. Resolution WHA 56.19 Prevention and control of influenza pandemics and annual epidemics. In: Fifty-sixth World Health Assembly, Geneva 19-28 May, 2003.
31. Resolution WHA 58.5 Prevention and control of influenza pandemics and annual epidemics. In: Fifty-eighth World Health Assembly, Geneva 16-25 May, 2005 (WHA58/2005/REC/1).
32. Resolution WHA 56.19 Prevention and control of influenza pandemics and annual epidemics. In: Fifty-sixth World Health Assembly, Geneva 19-28 May, 2003 and Resolution WHA 58.5 Prevention and control of influenza pandemics and annual epidemics. In: Fifty-eighth World Health Assembly, Geneva 16-25 May, 2005 (WHA58/2005/REC/1).
33. Using current FAO and OIE guidelines: Avian influenza and the virus that causes it(ftp://ftp.fao.org/docrep/fao/010/a0632e/a0632e02.pdf accessed 8 October 2008), Terrestrial Animal Health Code 2008, Article 10.4.29, Surveillance strategies (http://www.oie.int/eng/normes/mcode/en_index.htm accessed 8 October 2008).

PHASES 1-3
SITUATION MONITORING AND ASSESSMENT

WHO ACTIONS

- Collect, synthesize, and disseminate information on the global human influenza situation in collaboration with partners.
- Provide guidance and tools for detection, investigation, rapid risk assessment, reporting and ongoing evaluation of clusters of influenza-like illness.
- Provide support to countries with human cases of influenza caused by viruses with pandemic potential to assist in establishing facts and fully characterizing cases.
- Develop tools to estimate seasonal and pandemic influenza disease burden.[30]
- Establish joint initiatives for closer collaboration with national and international partners, including FAO and the OIE, in the early detection, reporting and investigation of influenza outbreaks of pandemic potential, and in coordinating research on the human-animal interface.[31]
- Establish global case definitions for reporting by countries of human cases of influenza caused by viruses with pandemic potential.
- Strengthen the Global Influenza Surveillance Network and other laboratories to increase capacity for influenza surveillance.[32]
- Provide diagnostic reagents to national influenza reference centres for identification of the new strain.
- Coordinate collection and testing of strains for possible vaccine production and antiviral susceptibility.

NATIONAL ACTIONS

- Develop national surveillance systems to collect up-to-date clinical, virological, and epidemiological information on trends in human infection with seasonal influenza viruses, which will also help to estimate additional needs during a pandemic.
- Detect animal[33] and human infections with animal influenza viruses, identify potential animal sources of human infection, assess the risk of transmission to humans, and communicate this information to WHO and relevant partners.
- Detect and investigate unusual clusters of influenza-like respiratory illness or deaths and assess for human-to-human transmission.
- Characterize and share both animal and human influenza virus isolates and associated information with relevant international agencies, such as WHO, FAO and OIE, to develop diagnostic reagents, candidate vaccine viruses, and monitor antiviral resistance.
- Strengthen the national laboratories in influenza diagnostic capabilities.

34. Resolution WHA 56.19 Prevention and control of influenza pandemics and annual epidemics. In: Fifty-sixth World Health Assembly, Geneva 19-28 May, 2003 and Resolution WHA 58.5 Prevention and control of influenza pandemics and annual epidemics. In: Fifty-eighth World Health Assembly, Geneva 16-25 May, 2005 (WHA58/2005/REC/1).

35. Prequalification. World Health Organization (http://www.who.int/hiv/amds/prequalification/en/ accessed 11 February, 2009).

36. Essential medecines list and WHO model formulary. World Health Organization (http://www.who.int/selection_medicines/list/en/ accessed 11 February, 2009).

37. Resolution WHA 58.5 Prevention and control of influenza pandemics and annual epidemics. In: Fifty-eighth World Health Assembly, Geneva 16-25 May, 2005 (WHA58/2005/REC/1).

38. Resolution WHA 60.28 Pandemic influenza preparedness: sharing of influenza viruses and access to vaccines and other benefits In: Sixtieth World Health Assembly, Geneva 14-23 May, 2007 (WHASS1/2006-WHA60/2007/REC/1).

39. Avian influenza: guidelines, recommendations, descriptions. World Health Organiztion (http://www.who.int/csr/disease/avian_influenza/guidelinestopics/en/index.html accessed 11 February, 2009).

40. Infection prevention and control of epidemic- and pandemic-prone acute respiratory diseases in health care, WHO Interim Guidelines. Geneva, World Health Organization 2007. (WHO/CDS/EPR/2007.6).

41. Infection prevention and control of epidemic- and pandemic-prone acute respiratory diseases in health care, WHO Interim Guidelines. Geneva, World Health Organization 2007. (WHO/CDS/EPR/2007.6).

42. Communicable disease alert and response for mass gatherings. Geneva, World Health Organization, 2008 (WHO/HSE/EPR/2008.8).

43. Resolution WHA 56.19 Prevention and control of influenza pandemics and annual epidemics. In: Fifty-sixth World Health Assembly, Geneva 19-28 May, 2003.

44. Resolution WHA 56.19 Prevention and control of influenza pandemics and annual epidemics. In: Fifty-sixth World Health Assembly, Geneva 19-28 May, 2003.

45. Currently there are no WHO recommendations either supporting or opposing the stockpiling of new influenza vaccines for use either prior to a pandemic or during its early stages.

46. Guidelines for the deployment of a pandemic influenza vaccine (to be published in 2009). World Health Organization 2009.

47. Pneumococcal conjugate vaccine for childhood immunization - WHO position paper. Weekly Epidemiological Record, No. 12, 2007, 82:93-104.

PHASES 1-3
REDUCING THE SPREAD OF DISEASE

WHO ACTIONS

- Promote agreements for international technical assistance and resource mobilization to resource-poor countries with foci of influenza activity.

Preventing human influenza infection from animals

- Activate joint mechanisms for actions with other organizations (e.g. FAO, OIE) to control disease in animals and to implement prevention measures.
- Encourage dissemination of information on spread in animals and interspecies transfers.

Individual/Societal level measures

- Provide guidance on measures to reduce the spread of influenza disease (social distancing and use of pharmaceuticals) and develop tools to estimate their public health value.[34]
- Periodically reassess and modify recommended interventions in consultation with appropriate partners, including those not in the health-care sector, regarding acceptability, effectiveness and feasibility.

Antivirals

- Develop principles to guide national recommendations for use of antivirals (for prophylaxis and treatment).
- Manage WHO strategic global stockpile of antivirals and develop standard operating procedures for rapid deployment.
- Increase global antiviral availability by using UN/WHO mechanism such as the prequalification programme[35] and the Essential Medicines List.[36]

Vaccines

- Develop principles to guide national recommendations for use of seasonal and pandemic vaccines.
- Support strain characterization and development and distribution of vaccine prototype strains for possible vaccine production.
- Review and update WHO recommendations for pandemic vaccine use.
- Provide technical support, capacity building and technology transfer for influenza vaccines and diagnostics to developing countries.[37]
- Formulate mechanisms and guidelines to promote fair and equitable distribution of pandemic influenza vaccines.[38]
- Manage an international stockpile of H5N1 vaccine for use in countries in need.

NATIONAL ACTIONS

- Identify, regularly brief, and train key personnel to be mobilized as part of a multisectoral expert response team for animal or human influenza outbreaks of pandemic potential.

Preventing human influenza infection from animals[39]

- Reduce infection risk in those involved in responding to animal outbreaks (education and training regarding the potential risk of transmission; correct use of personal protective equipment; making antivirals available if indicated by the risk assessment).
- Recommend measures to reduce human contact with potentially infected animals.
- Control potentially contaminated environments such as wet markets and ponds with free grazing ducks.
- In conjunction with animal health authorities, establish national guidance on food safety, safe agricultural practices, and public health issues related to influenza infection among animals.

Individual / household level measures

- Promote hand and respiratory hygiene.[40]
- Develop infection control guidance for household settings.[41]
- Develop plans to provide necessary support for ill persons isolated at home and their household contacts.

Societal level measures

- Establish protocols to suspend classes, especially in the event of a severe pandemic or if there is disproportionate or severe disease in children.
- Promote development of mitigation strategies for public and private sector workplaces (such as adjusting working patterns and practices).
- Promote reduction of unnecessary travel and overcrowding of mass transport systems.
- Develop a framework to facilitate decision-making for cancellation /restriction of mass gatherings at the time of the pandemic.[42]

International travel measures

- Develop capacities for emergency public health actions at designated points of entry in accordance with IHR (2005) Annex 1 B.2.

Antivirals and other pharmaceuticals

- Estimate and prioritize antiviral requirements for treatment and prophylaxis during a pandemic.
- Develop mechanisms and procedures to select, procure, stockpile, distribute, and deliver antivirals based on national goals and resources.
- Plan for the increased need for antibiotics, antipyretics, hydration, oxygen, and ventilation support within the context of national clinical management strategies.
- Assess effectiveness and safety of antiviral therapy using standardized protocols when possible.

Vaccines

- For countries not using seasonal influenza vaccine, document the disease burden and economic impact of seasonal influenza and develop a national vaccine, policy if indicated.[43]
- For countries using seasonal influenza vaccine, work to increase seasonal influenza vaccine coverage levels of all high risk people. [44]
- Establish goals and priorities for the use of pandemic influenza vaccines.[45]
- Develop a deployment plan to deliver pandemic influenza vaccines to national distribution points within seven days from when the vaccine is available to the national government.[46]
- Consider the feasibility of using pneumococcal vaccines as part of the routine immunization program in accordance with WHO guidelines.[47]

1-3 PREDOMINANTLY ANIMAL INFECTIONS; FEW HUMAN INFECTIONS

48.Infection prevention and control of epidemic- and pandemic-prone acute respiratory diseases in health care, WHO Interim Guidelines. Geneva, World Health Organization 2007. (WHO/CDS/EPR/2007.6).
49.Infection prevention and control of epidemic- and pandemic-prone acute respiratory diseases in health care, WHO Interim Guidelines. Geneva, World Health Organization 2007. (WHO/CDS/EPR/2007.6).
50.Collecting, preserving and shipping specimens for the diagnosis of avian influenza A(H5N1) virus infection, Guide for field operations. World Health Organization 2006 (WHO/CDS/EPR/ARO/2006.1) .

PHASES 1-3
CONTINIUITY OF HEALTH CARE PROVISION

WHO ACTIONS

- Provide guidance for appropriate infection control, laboratory biosafety and clinical management in health care and social settings, and in care facilities.
- Establish regional clinical advisory network for timely distribution and collection of important clinical information, identify knowledge gaps, and develop standardized clinical protocols.
- Assist national health care delivery authorities in identifying priority needs and response strategies, and assessing preparedness (e.g. through developing checklists, model pandemic preparedness plans, training and table-top exercises).
- Develop guidance for remote, resource-poor communities on home-based care of patients during an influenza pandemic.

NATIONAL ACTIONS

- Identify priorities and response strategies for public and private health care systems for triage, surge capacity, and human and material resource management.
- Review and update continuity of health care provision strategies at national and sub national levels.
- Develop strategies, plans, and training to enable all health care workers, including community level workers, to respond during animal outbreaks and a pandemic.
- Develop case-finding, treatment, and management protocols, and algorithms.
- Develop national infection control guidance.[48]
- Estimate and plan for procurement and distribution of personal protective equipment for protection of workers.[49]
- Develop and implement routine laboratory biosafety and safe specimen-handling and shipping policies and procedures.[50]
- Explore ways to provide drugs and medical care free of charge (or cover by insurance) to encourage prompt reporting and treatment of human cases caused by an animal influenza virus or virus with pandemic potential.
- Develop the capacity for the rapid deployment of diagnostic tests once available.
- Assess health system capacity to detect and contain outbreaks of human influenza disease in hospital settings.

51. World Health Organization Outbreak Communication Planning Guide. World Health Organization 2008. ISBN 978 92 4 159744 9.

PHASES 1-3
COMMUNICATIONS

WHO ACTIONS

- Update national and international authorities, other partners /stakeholders, and the public, with current information on risks, sources, personal safety, and ways of mitigation of influenza pandemics.
- Maintain formal communication channels among Member States, other international organizations, key stakeholders, and technical/professional associations to facilitate information sharing and coordination.
- Increase the familiarity of news media with WHO activities, operations, and decision-making related to influenza and other epidemic-prone diseases.
- Develop feedback mechanisms to identify emerging public concerns, address rumours, and correct misinformation.
- Support Member States' communication efforts during a pandemic by providing material and technical guidance.[51]

NATIONAL ACTIONS

- Establish an emergency communications committee with all necessary standard operating procedures to ensure a streamlined, expedited dissemination of communications products.
- Update leadership and other relevant sectors regarding global and national pandemic influenza risk status.
- Build effective relations with key journalists and other communications channels to familiarize them with influenza and pandemic related issues.
- Develop effective dialogue and listening mechanisms with the general public.
- Develop effective communication strategies and messages to inform, educate, and communicate with individuals and families so they are better able to take appropriate actions before, during, and after a pandemic.
- Initiate public health education campaigns in coordination with other relevant authorities on individual-level infection control measures.
- Increase public awareness of measures that may be available to reduce the spread of pandemic influenza.
- Create messages and feedback mechanisms targeted towards hard-to-reach, disadvantaged, or minority groups.
- Test communications procedures through exercises.
- Update communications strategies as feedback from the general public and stakeholder organizations is collected and analysed.

4 SUSTAINED HUMAN-TO-HUMAN TRANSMISSION

B. PHASE 4

An important goal during WHO pandemic Phase 4 is to contain the new virus within a limited area or delay its spread to gain time to implement interventions, including the use of vaccines.

PHASE 4
PLANNING AND COORDINATION

WHO ACTIONS

- Consult with the affected country and external experts on the decision to launch a rapid containment operation.
- Provide ongoing advice to the affected country on the management of the containment operation.
- Coordinate the international response to rapid containment, including the deployment of international field teams as requested and necessary.
- Mobilize and dispatch resources (e.g. antivirals from the global stockpile, other materials and logistics) for rapid containment.
- Mobilize financial resources for a rapid containment operation as needed and encourage the provision of international assistance to resource-poor countries.
- Initiate planning and actions to switch from seasonal to pandemic vaccine production.

NATIONAL ACTIONS

FOR AFFECTED COUNTRIES
- Direct and coordinate rapid pandemic containment activities in collaboration with WHO to limit the spread of human infection.
- Activate national emergency and crisis committee(s) and national command, control, and coordination mechanisms for emergency operations.
- Activate procedures to access and mobilize additional human and material resources.
- Deploy operational and logistics response teams.
- Identify needs for international assistance.
- Designate special status as needed (such as declaring a state of emergency) to facilitate rapid containment interventions.
- Provide regular updates on the evolving situation to WHO as required under IHR (2005) and to other partners to facilitate coordination of response.
- Encourage cross-border collaboration with surrounding countries through information sharing and coordination of responses.
- Activate pandemic contingency plans for all sectors as deemed critical for the provision of essential services.
- Finalize preparations for a possible pandemic including procurement plans for essential pharmaceuticals.

COUNTRIES NOT YET AFFECTED
- Finalize preparations for a possible pandemic by activating internal organizational arrangements within the command-and-control mechanism and mobilizing staffing surge capacity in critical services.
- Respond, if possible, to requests for international assistance organized by WHO.

52. WHO Interim planning guidance for rapid containment of the initial emergence of pandemic influenza. (http://www.who.int/csr/disease/avian_influenza/guidelines/draftprotocol/en/index.html accessed 10 February 2009).
53. WHO Interim planning guidance for rapid containment of the initial emergence of pandemic influenza. (http://www.who.int/csr/disease/avian_influenza/guidelines/draftprotocol/en/index.html accessed 10 February 2009) and WHO Global Surveillance for Pandemic Influenza, World Health Organization 2009 (to be published 2009 http://www.who.int/csr/disease/influenza/).

PHASE 4
SITUATION MONITORING AND ASSESSMENT

WHO ACTIONS

- Provide support to national authorities and facilitate assessment of the extent of human-to human transmission with on-site evaluation.
- Refine case definition for global reporting.
- Recommend strategies for national authorities to enhance surveillance in affected areas.
- Coordinate collection and testing of specimens and/or strains to develop diagnostic reagents, prototype vaccines, and for antiviral susceptibility.
- Coordinate with national authorities to monitor containment measures.

NATIONAL ACTIONS

FOR AFFECTED COUNTRIES

- Enhance surveillance to rapidly detect, investigate, and report new cases and clusters.[52]
- Collect specimens for testing and virological characterization using protocols and procedures developed in collaboration with WHO.
- Share specimens and/or strains to develop diagnostic reagents and prototype vaccines and for antiviral susceptibility.
- Collect more detailed epidemiological and clinical data as time and resources permit.[53]
- To the extent possible, monitor compliance, safety, and effectiveness of mitigation measures and share findings with the international community and WHO.

FOR COUNTRIES NOT YET AFFECTED

- Enhance virological and epidemiological surveillance to detect possible cases and clusters, especially if sharing extensive travel or trade links with affected areas.
- Report any suspect cases to national authorities and WHO.

4 SUSTAINED HUMAN-TO-HUMAN TRANSMISSION

54. It exit screening is implemented, it should be considered as a time-limited intervention and the isolation and treatment of cases and quarantine of contacts resulting from screening must be carried out in accordance with IHR (2005).

55. WHO Interim Protocol: Rapid operations to contain the initial emergence of pandemic influenza. (http://www.who.int/csr/disease/avian_influenza/guidelines/draftprotocol/en/index.html accessed 8 October 2008).

56. Recommended interventions to reduce the spread of disease during pandemic influenza. World Health Organization 2009 (to be published 2009 http://www.who.int/csr/disease/influenza/).

57. Infection prevention and control of epidemic- and pandemic-prone acute respiratory diseases in health care, WHO Interim Guidelines. Geneva, World Health Organization 2007.(WHO/CDS/EPR/2007.6).

PHASE 4
REDUCING THE SPREAD OF DISEASE

WHO ACTIONS

- Assist the affected country in undertaking rapid pandemic containment operations coordinating international collaboration.
- Dispatch antivirals from the WHO stockpile to the affected country, to be used in rapid containment operations.
- Develop up-to-date vaccine prototype strains.
- Collaborate with national authorities in determining possible use of a potentially effective vaccine during rapid containment operations.
- Update guidance for optimal use of pandemic vaccines when available.

NATIONAL ACTIONS

ALL COUNTRIES
International travel measures

- Consider implementing exit screening as part of the early global response (i.e. first few affected countries).[54]
- Provide advice to travellers.

AFFECTED COUNTRIES

- Undertake rapid pandemic containment[55] operations in collaboration with WHO and the international community.
- Request and distribute antivirals from the WHO global stockpile and/or other national or regional stockpiles for treatment of cases and prophylaxis of all persons in the designated areas.
- Consider deploying pandemic vaccine if available.
- Implement individual/household and societal-level disease control measures.[56]
- Limit all non-essential movement of persons in and out of the designated containment area(s) and implement screening procedures at transit points.

COUNTRIES NOT YET AFFECTED

- Reassess the capacity to implement mitigation measures to reduce the spread of pandemic influenza.
- Distribute stockpiles of pharmaceuticals and other materials according to national plans.
- Use appropriate individual/household disease control measures for suspect cases and their contacts.[57]

WHO ACTIONS	NATIONAL ACTIONS

WHO ACTIONS

- Coordinate and support collection of clinical data to reassess clinical management guidelines and protocols.
- Update guidelines for clinical management and infection control as necessary.
- Update guidelines for biosafety in laboratories as necessary.

NATIONAL ACTIONS

AFFECTED COUNTRIES
- Provide guidance to health care workers to consider influenza infection in patients with respiratory illness and to test and report suspect cases.
- Implement appropriate infection control measures and issue personal protective equipment as needed.
- Activate contingency plans for responding to the possible overload of health and laboratory facilities to deal with potential staff shortages.
- Activate alternative strategies for case isolation and management as needed.

COUNTRIES NOT YET AFFECTED
- Activate pandemic contingency planning arrangements for the health sector.
- Advise health care workers to consider the possibility of influenza infection in patients with respiratory illness, especially those with travel or other contact with persons in the affected country(ies).

4 SUSTAINED HUMAN-TO-HUMAN TRANSMISSION

WHO ACTIONS

- Update national and international authorities, other partners, stakeholders, and the public on global epidemiological situation, disease characteristics, and the containment efforts.
- Issue updates on the effectiveness of various public health measures as data become available.
- Coordinate and disseminate relevant public health messages using various channels (WHO website, published material, press conferences, and the media).
- Work with partners to promote consistent messages.

NATIONAL ACTIONS

FOR ALL COUNTRIES

- Activate communications mechanisms to ensure widest possible dissemination of information.
- Update and disseminate "Talking Points" so that all spokespeople convey consistent information.
- Conduct frequent and pre-announced public briefings through popular media outlets such as the web, television, radio, and press conferences to counter panic and dispel rumours.

FOR AFFECTED COUNTRIES

- Regularly communicate via established mechanisms:
  - What is known and not known about the virus, the state of the outbreak, use and effectiveness of measures and likely next steps.
  - The importance of limiting all non-essential movement of persons in and out of the designated containment area(s) and relevant screening procedures at transit points.
  - The importance of compliance with recommended measures to stop further spread of the disease.
  - How to obtain medicines, essential services and supplies in the containment area(s).
- Gather feedback from the general public, vulnerable populations and at-risk groups on attitudes towards the recommended measures and barriers affecting their willingness or ability to comply. Incorporate the findings into communication and health education campaigns targeted to the specific groups.
- Collaborate with surrounding countries on information sharing.

C. PHASES 5-6

During Phases 5-6 (*pandemic*), actions shift from preparedness to response at a global level. The goal of recommended actions during these phases is to reduce the impact of the pandemic on society.

26. Resolution WHA 56.19 Prevention and control of influenza pandemics and annual epidemics. In: Fifty-sixth World Health Assembly, Geneva 19-28 May, 2003
27. Resolution WHA 56.19 Prevention and control of influenza pandemics and annual epidemics. In: Fifty-sixth World Health Assembly, Geneva 19-28 May, 2003.
28. Resolution WHA 56.19 Prevention and control of influenza pandemics and annual epidemics. In: Fifty-sixth World Health Assembly, Geneva 19-28 May, 2003.
29. Ethical considerations in developing a public health response to pandemic influenza (WHO/CDS/EPR/GIP/2007.2), World Health Organization, 2007.

PHASES 5-6
PLANNING AND COORDINATION

WHO ACTIONS

- Encourage international assistance to resource-poor countries and/or seriously affected countries.
- Interact with international organizations and agencies inside and outside of the health sector to coordinate interventions.

NATIONAL ACTIONS

AFFECTED COUNTRIES
- Maintain trust across all agencies and organizations and with the public through a commitment to transparency and credible actions.
- Designate special status as needed, such as declaring a state of emergency.
- Provide leadership and coordination to multisectoral resources to mitigate the societal and economic impact of a pandemic.
- Work for rational, ethical, and transparent access to resources.
- Assess if external assistance is required to meet humanitarian needs.

COUNTRIES NOT YET AFFECTED
- Finalize preparations for an imminent pandemic, including activation of crisis committee(s) and national command and control systems.
- Update, if necessary, national guidance and recommendations taking into account information from affected countries.

PHASES 5-6

5-6 PANDEMIC

WIDESPREAD HUMAN INFECTION

58. Global surveillance during an influenza pandemic, World Health Organization 2009 (to be published 2009 to http://www.who.int/csr/disease/influenza/).

PHASES 5-6
SITUATION MONITORING AND ASSESSMENT

WHO ACTIONS

- Coordinate the assessment and monitoring of the disease characteristics and severity, and provide guidance accordingly.
- Monitor the global spread of disease and possible changes in epidemiological, clinical, and virological aspects of infection, including antiviral drug resistance.
- Support affected Member States as much as possible in confirming the spread of human infections and assessing the epidemiological situation.

NATIONAL ACTIONS

AFFECTED COUNTRIES

Pandemic disease surveillance[58]

- Undertake a comprehensive assessment of the earliest cases of pandemic influenza.
- Document the evolving pandemic including geographical spread, trends, and impact.
- Document any changes in epidemiological and clinical features of the pandemic virus.
- Maintain adequate virological surveillance to detect antigenic and genetic changes, as well as changes in antiviral susceptibility and pathogenicity.
- Modify national case definitions and update clinical and laboratory algorithms for diagnosis, as necessary.

Monitoring and assessment of the impact of the pandemic

- Monitor essential health-related resources such as: medical supplies; antivirals, vaccines and other pharmaceuticals; health care worker availability, hospital occupancy/availability; use of alternative health facilities, laboratory material stocks; and mortuary capacity.
- Monitor and assess national impact using criteria such as workplace and school absenteeism, regions affected, groups most affected, and essential worker availability.
- Assess the uptake and impact of implemented mitigation measures.
- Forecast economic impact of the pandemic, if possible.

59. Assuming a PHEIC has been determined to be occurring as defined by IHR (2005)

60. Especially if non-pandemic strains are still circulating.

61. If medical masks are available and the training on their correct use is feasible, they may be considered for symptomatic persons and susceptible caregivers in household settings when close contact can not be avoided.

62. Infection prevention and control of epidemic- and pandemic-prone acute respiratory diseases in health care, WHO Interim Guidelines. Geneva, World Health Organization 2007. (WHO/CDS/EPR/2007.6)

63. Symptomatic people should self-isolate and avoid using public transport. There is, however, insufficient evidence to date to either support or oppose the closure or restriction of mass transport systems as a measure to reduce disease transmission in the community.

64. If a country decides to cancel, restrict or modify all or certain mass gatherings, this decision should be based on the nature of the gathering and on local disease levels, and should only be implemented once the disease is present in the community.

65. It exit screening is implemented, it should be considered as a time-limited intervention and the isolation and treatment of cases and quarantine of contacts resulting from screening must be carried out in accordance with IHR (2005).

66. It entry screening is implemented, it should be considered as a time-limited intervention and the isolation and treatment of cases and quarantine of contacts resulting from screening must be carried out in accordance with IHR (2005).

PHASES 5-6
REDUCING THE SPREAD OF DISEASE

WHO ACTIONS

- Consider and issue any new or revised Temporary Recommendations under IHR (2005), including advice from Emergency Committee as appropriate.[59]
- Facilitate assessment of interventions and update recommendations if needed.
- Facilitate assessment of antiviral susceptibility, effectiveness, and safety.
- Make recommendations for pandemic vaccine composition[60] and switch to pandemic vaccine production if not previously done.
- Facilitate development of national guidelines for national authorities to conduct targeted vaccination campaigns if pandemic vaccine is available.

NATIONAL ACTIONS

ALL COUNTRIES
International travel measures
- Take into account WHO guidance and information when issuing international travel advisories and health alerts.

AFFECTED COUNTRIES
Individual/household level measures
- Advise people with acute respiratory illness to stay at home and to minimize their contact with household members and others.
- Advise household contacts to minimize their level of interaction outside the home and to isolate themselves at the first sign of any symptoms of influenza.
- Provide infection control guidance for household caregivers[61] taking into account the WHO Guidance.[62]

Societal level measures
- Implement social distancing measures as indicated in national plans, such as class suspensions and adjusting working patterns.
- Encourage reduction in travel and crowding of the mass transport system.[63]
- Assess and determine if cancellation, restriction, or modification of mass gatherings is indicated.[64]

International travel measures
- Consider implementing exit screening as part of the early global response (i.e. first few affected countries).[65]
- Provide advice to travellers.

Pharmaceutical measures
- Distribute antivirals, and other medical supplies in accordance with national plans.
- Implement vaccine procurement plans.
- Plan for vaccine distribution and accelerate preparations for mass vaccination campaigns.
- Modify/adapt antiviral and vaccine strategies based on monitoring and surveillance information.
- Implement medical prophylaxis campaigns for antivirals and/or vaccines according to priority status and availability in accordance with national plans.
- Monitor safety and efficacy of pharmaceutical interventions to the extent possible and monitor supply.

COUNTRIES NOT YET AFFECTED
- Be prepared to implement planned interventions to reduce the spread of pandemic disease.
- Update recommendations on the use of planned interventions based on experience and information from affected countries.
- Implement distribution and deployment plans for pharmaceuticals, and other resources as required.
- Consider implementing entry screening at international borders.[66]

WHO recognizes individual country considerations will affect national decisions, but, in general, does not encourage:
- **Pandemic-related international border closures for people and/or cargo.**
- **General disinfection of the environment during a pandemic.**
- **The use of masks in the community by well persons.**
- **The restriction of travel within national borders during a pandemic, with the exception of a globally led rapid response and containment operation, or in rare instances where clear geographical and other barriers exist.**

5-6 PANDEMIC
WIDESPREAD HUMAN INFECTION

WHO ACTIONS	NATIONAL ACTIONS
• Coordinate response with other international organizations. • Provide guidance to national authorities in assisting clinicians in recognition, diagnosis, and reporting of cases and other critical issues as needed.	• Implement pandemic contingency plans for full mobilization of health systems, facilities, and workers at national and sub-national levels. • Implement and adjust the triage system as necessary. • Enhance infection control practices in healthcare and laboratory settings and distribute personal protective equipment in accordance with national plans. • Provide medical and non-medical support for patients and their contacts in households and alternative facilities if needed. • Provide social and psychological support for health care workers, patients, and communities. • Implement corpse management procedures as necessary. **FOR COUNTRIES NOT YET AFFECTED** • Prepare to switch to pandemic working arrangements.

WHO ACTIONS	NATIONAL ACTIONS
• Update national authorities, other partners and stakeholders, and the public on global situation, trends, epidemiological characteristics, and recommended measures. • Continue to work with partners to promote consistent messages.	• Regularly update the public on what is known and unknown about the pandemic disease, including transmission patterns, clinical severity, treatment, and prophylaxis options. • Provide regular communications to address societal concerns, such as the disruption to travel, border closures, schools, or the economy or society in general. • Regularly update the public on sources of emergency medical care, resources for dealing with urgent non-pandemic health care needs, and resources for self-care of medical conditions.

THE POST-PEAK PERIOD

D. THE POST-PEAK PERIOD

The overall goal of actions during the post-peak period is to address the health and social impact of the pandemic, as well as to prepare for possible future pandemic waves.

THE POST-PEAK PERIOD
PLANNING AND COORDINATION

WHO ACTIONS	NATIONAL ACTIONS
• Identify lessons learned for immediate application, as well as for future needs.	• Determine the need for additional resources and capacities during possible future pandemic waves.
	• Begin rebuilding of essential services
	• Address the psychological impacts of the pandemic, especially on the health workforce.
	• Consider offering assistance to countries with ongoing pandemic activity.
	• Review the status of and replenish national, local, and household stockpiles and supplies.
	• Review and revise national plans.

THE POST-PEAK PERIOD
SITUATION MONITORING AND ASSESSMENT

WHO ACTIONS	NATIONAL ACTIONS
• Assist countries in estimating national impact.	• Activate the surveillance activities required to detect subsequent pandemic waves.
• Continue global situation monitoring for global spread and national trends.	• Evaluate the resources needed to monitor subsequent waves.
• Review lessons learned and make adjustments in surveillance guidelines and tools for countries.	
• Assess and monitor the type and pathogenicity of circulating influenza viruses.	

THE POST-PEAK PERIOD

POSSIBILITY OF RECURRENT EVENTS

REDUCING THE SPREAD OF DISEASE

WHO ACTIONS

NATIONAL ACTIONS

- Facilitate evaluation of interventions.

- Evaluate the effectiveness of the measures used and update guidelines, protocols, and algorithms accordingly.
- Continue with vaccination programmes in accordance with national plans, priorities, and vaccine availability.

CONTINUITY OF HEALTH CARE PROVISION

WHO ACTIONS

NATIONAL ACTIONS

- Update guidance to national authorities to optimize use of scarce facilities.

- Ensure that health care personnel have the opportunity for rest and recuperation.
- Restock medications and supplies and service and renew essential equipment.
- Review and, if necessary, revise pandemic preparedness and response plans in anticipation of possible future pandemic wave(s).
- Revise case definitions, treatment protocols, and algorithms as required.

COMMUNICATIONS

WHO ACTIONS

NATIONAL ACTIONS

- Regularly update the public and other stakeholders on any changes to the status of the pandemic.
- Urge Member States, partners, and other stakeholders to make adjustments to their communications plans and systems.

- Regularly update the public and other stakeholders on any changes to the status of the pandemic.
- Communicate to the public the ongoing need for vigilance and disease-prevention efforts to prevent any upswing in disease levels.
- Continue to update the health sector on new information or other changes that affect disease status, signs and symptoms, or case definitions, protocols and algorithms.

THE POST-PANDEMIC PERIOD

E. THE POST-PANDEMIC PERIOD

The goal of activities during the post-pandemic period is to address the long-term health and social impact of the pandemic, as well as to restore normal health and social functions.

THE POST-PANDEMIC PERIOD
PLANNING AND COORDINATION

WHO ACTIONS	NATIONAL ACTIONS
• Facilitate implementation of lessons learned for immediate application, as well as for future needs.	• Evaluate the effectiveness of specific responses and interventions and share findings with the international community. • Review the lessons learned and apply to national emergency preparedness and response programmes. • Revise national and sub-national pandemic preparedness and response plans.

THE POST-PANDEMIC PERIOD
SITUATION MONITORING AND ASSESSMENT

WHO ACTIONS	NATIONAL ACTIONS
• Report on the global situation. • Review lessons learned and make adjustments in surveillance guidelines and tools for countries.	• Collect and analyse available data to evaluate the epidemiological, clinical, and virological characteristics of the pandemic. • Review and revise situation monitoring and assessment tools for the next pandemic and other public health emergencies. • Resume seasonal influenza surveillance incorporating the pandemic virus subtype as part of routine surveillance.

THE POST-PANDEMIC PERIOD
REDUCING THE SPREAD OF DISEASE

WHO ACTIONS	NATIONAL ACTIONS

• Provide technical support to Member States, as requested, to evaluate the impact of the pandemic on the country and the effectiveness and impact of interventions utilized during the pandemic.	• Conduct a thorough evaluation of individual, household, and societal interventions implemented.
	• Conduct a thorough evaluation of all the pharmaceutical interventions used, including:
	  • antiviral effectiveness, safety, and resistance; and
	  • vaccine coverage, effectiveness, and safety.
	• Review and update relevant guidelines as necessary.
	• Continue with vaccination programmes in accordance with national plans, priorities, and vaccine availability.

THE POST-PANDEMIC PERIOD

DISEASE ACTIVITY AT SEASONAL LEVELS

CONTINUITY OF HEALTH CARE PROVISION

WHO ACTIONS

- Utilize existing clinical networks to review clinical information and effectiveness and safety of clinical interventions; advise on knowledge gaps and research needs.
- Review and revise relevant guidance.

NATIONAL ACTIONS

- Collect and analyse available data to evaluate the response of the health system to the pandemic.
- Review the lessons learned and share experiences with the international community.
- Amend plans and procedures to include lessons learned.
- As needed, provide psychosocial services to facilitate individual and community-level recovery.

COMMUNICATIONS

WHO ACTIONS

- Evaluate communications response during previous phases; review lessons learned.
- Ensure that lessons learned are incorporated into revised and improved communications plans of all stakeholders, ready for use in the next pandemic/major public health event.
- Continue to work with Member States to increase the effectiveness of national communications activities.

NATIONAL ACTIONS

- Publicly acknowledge the contributions of all communities and sectors.
- Communicate to the public and other stakeholders the lessons learned about the effectiveness of responses during the pandemic and how the gaps that were discovered will be addressed.
- Encourage stakeholders across all sectors, public and private, to revise their pandemic and emergency plans based upon the lessons learned.
- Extend communications planning and activities to cover other epidemic diseases and use the principles of risk communications to build the capacity to dialogue with the public on all health matters of potential concern to them.
- Improve and adjust communications plan in readiness for the next major public health event.

This annex provides some parameters to be considered by national authorities in planning for pandemic influenza.

ANNEX 1 - PLANNING ASSUMPTIONS

GENERAL GUIDANCE IN PANDEMIC INFLUENZA PREPAREDNESS PLANNING ASSUMPTIONS

Planning for a future influenza pandemic is difficult in part because many important features of the next pandemic are not known. In this situation, assumptions relating to the epidemiology of influenza are needed to make decisions in public health planning, as well as estimating required resources.

This annex provides some parameters to be considered by national authorities in planning for pandemic influenza. These assumptions are based on information known at the time of publication about seasonal influenza, avian influenza, and past influenza pandemics.

These data should not be taken as predictions of how the next influenza pandemic will spread and its resulting impact. Features of the next pandemic will not be uniform worldwide. The characteristics and impacts of past pandemics have varied between countries and within an individual country. These differences are most likely attributable to both the characteristics of the pandemic virus and the ability of the country to respond to the disease.

It is beyond the scope of this Annex to provide a comprehensive review of the epidemiology of influenza. It will be updated as new scientific data become available that significantly change these assumptions. Key references are provided for readers to review the existing literature.

1. Modes of transmission

Suggested assumptions

- Modes of virus transmission of pandemic influenza are expected to be similar to those of seasonal influenza: via the large droplet or contact (either direct or indirect) route, with a contribution by particle airborne route, or a combination of both.
- The relative contribution and clinical importance of potentially different modes of transmission of influenza are unknown. However, epidemiological patterns suggest that the spread of the virus is mostly through close contact via the droplet or contact route.

Implications

- Good hand hygiene, isolation of ill persons, and the use of personal protective equipment are important measures when caring for persons with influenza to decrease viral transmission.
- An airborne precaution room is not indicated for routine care. However, health care workers should wear eye protection, a gown, clean non-sterile gloves, and particulate respirators during the performance of aerosol generating procedures.

Scientific basis

- Droplet and contact transmission appear to be major routes of transmission for seasonal influenza (Brankston G et al, 2007; Bridges CB et al, 2003).
- However, data are insufficient to determine the relative importance of the different modes of transmission. In addition, there is lack of standardization and consensus about the technical definition (i.e., particle size) of an aerosol versus a droplet (Tellier R, 2006; Lemieux, C et al, 2007).
- Relative heat and humidity impact the efficiency of transmission of influenza via aerosol. Some have reported the lack of aerosol transmission at 30oC, while transmission via the contact route was equally efficient at 30oC and 20oC (Lowen AC et al. 2007; Lowen AC et al. 2008).
- Certain procedures performed in health care settings can create aerosols. Some of these procedures have been associated with a significant increase in the risk of disease transmission and have been termed "aerosol-generating procedures associated with pathogen transmission" (WHO, 2007). These procedures include intubation, cardiopulmonary resuscitation, bronchoscopy, autopsy, and surgery where high-speed devices are used (WHO, 2007).

Selected References

- Brankston G, Gitterman L, Hirji Z et al. **Transmission of influenza A in human beings**. Lancet Infect Dis. 2007;7(4):257-65.
- Bridges CB, Kuehnert MJ, Hal CB. **Transmission of Influenza: Implications for Control in Health Care Settings**. Clinl Infect Dis 2003;37:1094-1101.
- Lemieux C, Brankston G, Gitterman L et al. **Questioning aerosol transmission of influenza**. Emerg Inf Dis, 2007;13(1):173-174.
- Lowen AC, Mubareka S, Steel J et al. **Influenza virus transmission is dependent on relative humidity and temperature**. PLoS Pathog. 2007 Oct 19;3(10):1470-6.
- Lowen AC, Steel J, Mubareka S et al. **High temperature (30 degrees C) blocks aerosol but not contact transmission of influenza virus**. J Virol. 2008;82(11):5650-2.
- Tang JW, Li Y, Eames I et al. **Factors involved in the aerosol transmission of infection and control of ventilation in healthcare premises** J Hosp Infect. 2006 Oct;64(2):100-14.
- Tellier R. **Review of aerosol transmission of influenza A virus**. Emerg Inf Dis, 2006;12(11):1657-1662.

2. Incubation period and infectiousness of pandemic influenza

Suggested assumptions

- Incubation period: 1 - 3 days
- Latent period: 0.5 - 2 days
- Duration of infectiousness: About five days in adults and could be longer in children
- Basic reproduction number (R0): 1.5 - 2.0.

Implications

- The incubation period and the duration of infectiousness are useful for planning purposes regarding: length of isolation for cases; development of a definition for contacts of cases; and the length of quarantining contacts.
- A relatively short incubation period would make it difficult to stop the spread of pandemic influenza by contact tracing and quarantine.
- Viral shedding before symptoms develop would make it difficult to stop the spread of pandemic influenza solely by screening and isolating clinically ill persons.
- Once the pandemic begins, it will be important for countries to undertake surveillance and special studies to assess the incubation period and the duration of infectiousness of the pandemic virus.

Scientific basis

- An early study using Australian maritime statistics suggested that the mean incubation period of the 1918 pandemic influenza was 32.71 hours (1.4 days). (McKendrick and Morison as reviewed by Nishiura, 2007).
- A meta-analysis of 56 volunteer studies (Carrat et al, 2008) found that:
  - an increase in the average total symptoms score was noted by day 1 after inoculation, total scores peaked by day 2 and returned to baseline values by day 8;
  - viral shedding increased sharply between 0.5 and 1 days after challenge and consistently peaked on day 2 (mean generation time 2.5 days); the average duration of viral shedding was 4.8 days;
  - viral shedding curves and total symptom score curves showed similar shapes, although viral shedding preceded illness by 1 day.
- Longer durations of viral shedding are not rare. As reviewed by Carrat et al., in one study subgroup, five participants (20 percent) shed influenza B virus eight days after inoculation, while another study also reported nine days of shedding for influenza A/H3N2.
- Reasonable estimates of the basic reproduction number (R0) for past pandemic viruses as well as seasonal influenza viruses converge between 1.5 and 2.0 (Ferguson NM et al., 2005; Ferguson NM et al., 2006; Colliza V et al., 2007; Vynnycky E et al. 2007).
- The incubation period of H5N1 human cases (7 days or less; mostly 2 - 5 days) appears to be longer than that of seasonal influenza. In clusters in which limited human-to-human transmission has probably occurred, the incubation period appears to be approximately 3 - 5 days, although in one cluster it was estimated to be 8 - 9 days (WHO writing committee, 2008).
- Patients with influenza A (H5N1) disease may have detectable viral RNA in the respiratory tract for up to three weeks; data, however, are limited. (Reviewed by WHO writing committee, 2008; and Gambotto et al., 2007).

Selected References

- Carrat F, Vergu E, Ferguson NM et al. **Time Lines of Infection and Disease in Human Influenza: A Review of Volunteer Challenge Studies.** Am. J. Epidemiol., 2008;167:775-785.
- Colliza V, Barrat A, Barthelemy M et al. **Modelling the worldwide spread of pandemic influenza: baseline case and containment interventions.** PLoS Medicine, 2007;4(1):95-110.

- Ferguson NM, Cummings DAT, Cauchemez S et al. **Strategies for containing an emerging influenza pandemic in Southeast Asia.** Nature, 2005;437(8):209-214.
- Ferguson NM, Cummings DAT, Fraser C et al. **Strategies for mitigating an influenza pandemic.** Nature 2006;442:448-452.
- Gambotto A, Barratt-Boyes SM, de Jong MD et al. **Human infection with highly pathogenic H5N1 influenza virus.** Lancet 2007;371:1464-75.
- Nishiura H. **Early efforts in modeling the incubation period of infectious diseases with an acute course of illness.** Emerging Themes in Epidemiology, 2007;4:2.
- Vynnycky E, Trindall A, Mangtani P. **Estimates of the reproduction numbers of Spanish influenza using morbidity data.** International Journal of Epidemiology. 2007;36:881-889.
- Writing committee of the second WHO consultation on clinical aspect of human infection with avian influenza A(H5N1) virus. **Update on Avian Influenza A** (H5N1) **Virus Infection in Humans.** N Engl J Med 2008;358:261-73.

3. Symptom development and clinical attack rate

Suggested assumptions

- About two-thirds of people with pandemic influenza are expected to develop clinical symptoms.
- Uncomplicated clinical symptoms of pandemic influenza are expected to be similar to those of seasonal influenza: respiratory symptoms, fever and abrupt onset of muscle ache, and headache or backache.
- Averaged overall (across all age groups), population clinical attack rates are expected to be 25% to 45%.

Implications

- Existing clinical criteria for influenza-like illness can serve as the basis for pandemic disease surveillance. However, countries are encouraged to closely monitor the evolution of clinical characteristics of pandemic influenza and to facilitate refinement of a clinical case definition.
- Given influenza's usual nonspecific clinical presentations, pandemic surveillance should be supported by laboratory diagnosis. This is critical to confirm and comprehensively describe the first cases in each country.
- Because the number of ill persons may overwhelm the existing health care capacities, countries should plan for rapid scaling up of health care capacity and prioritization of limited resources.
- Wide variations in clinical attack rates among different age groups and localities have been observed with previous pandemics. Countries are encouraged to estimate clinical attack rates based on their own data and experiences.

Scientific basis

- A pooled analysis of 522 persons who were voluntarily infected with influenza reported the proportion of symptomatic infection (any symptoms) as 66.9% (95% CI: 58.3, 74.5). No significant differences were noted according to the virus type or the initial infectious dose (Carrat et al, 2008).

- A modelling study using 1957 pandemic data from the UK estimated that 60 - 65% of infected individuals experienced clinical symptoms (Vynnycky E et al., 2008).
- An analysis an influenza outbreak experience in an isolated island, Tristina da Cunha, in 1971 suggested that almost all susceptible persons developed symptomatic illness (Mathews JD et al., 2007).
- During the 1918 pandemic in the United States, influenza-like illness rates averaged 28%, with a low of 15% and a high of 50% (Frost WH, 1919). These data were based on house-to-house surveys.
- In one report, age-specific serological attack rates for the 1957 pandemic averaged 40%, with a low of 5% and a high of 70%. In contrast, a 20% serological attack rate was reported for the 1968 pandemic (Stuart-Harris CH, 1970).
- A retrospective questionnaire survey from one US city revealed the overall clinical attack rate during the 1968 pandemic was 39%; and it was similar among all age groups (Davis LE et al., 1970). Another serological survey found that about 25% (range of 21% to 27%) of children tested positive for antibodies to the influenza strain that circulated in 1968 (Chin J et al., 1974).
- Clinical attack rates calculated from an estimated basic reproduction number (R0) between 1.5 and 2.0 range from approximately 25% to 45% (Ferguson NM et al., 2005; Ferguson NM et al., 2006; Germann TC et al., 2006; Colliza V et al., 2007; Halloran ME et al., 2008).
- Gastrointestinal symptoms have been observed among patients with influenza A (H5N1), but have varied by clades (WHO writing committee, 2008).

Selected References

- Frost WH. **The epidemiology of influenza.** Pub Health Reports; 1919;34(33) (republished in Pub Health Report, 2006;121(S1):149-158).
- Stuart-Harris CH. **Pandemic influenza: an unresolved problem in prevention.** J Infect Dis, 1970;122:108-115.
- Davis LE, Caldwell GG, Lynch RE. **Hong Kong influenza: the epidemiologic features of a high school family study analyzed and compared with a similar study during the 1957 Asian influenza epidemic.** Amer J Epid, 1970;92:240-247.
- Chin J, Magoffin RL, Lennette EH. **The epidemiology of influenza in California, 1968-1973.** West J Med. 1974;121:94-99.
- Germann TC, Kadau K, Longini, IM Jr. et al. **Mitigation strategies for pandemic influenza in the United States.** PNAS, 2006;103(15):5935-5940.
- Halloran ME, Ferguson NM, Eubank S et al. **Modeling targeted layered containment of an influenza pandemic in the United States.** PNAS, 2008;105(12):4639-4644.
- Mathews JD, McCaw CT, McVernon et al. **A biological model for influenza transmission: pandemic planning implication of asymptomatic infection and immunity.** PLoS ONE, 2007;2(11):e1220.
- Vynnycky E, Edmunds WJ. **Analyses of the 1957 (Asian) influenza pandemic in the United Kingdom and the impact of school closures.** Epidemiol Infect. 2008;136(2):166-79.

4. Dynamics of the pandemic and its impact

Suggested assumptions

- An influenza pandemic can begin at any time of the year and any place in the world; it is expected to spread to the rest of the world within several weeks or months.
- Duration of a pandemic wave is expected to be from several weeks to a few months, but will likely vary from country to country; within a single country variations may be seen by community.
- Most communities are expected to experience multiple waves of a pandemic.
- Increased hospitalizations, excess mortality, and secondary complications are expected to vary widely among countries and communities. Vulnerable populations are expected to be affected more severely.
- Workplace absenteeism is expected to be higher than the estimated clinical attack rate.

Implications

- Each county should develop and strengthen its capacity to detect the early emergence of a potential pandemic event and to respond rapidly.
- Countries should guide their local governments and communities to develop their own pandemic influenza preparedness and response plans.
- Actions during the post-peak periods between pandemic waves should be considered in overall pandemic preparedness and response plans.
- Countries are encouraged to further estimate and prepare health care needs based on their own resources and experiences, with particular concern to vulnerable populations.
- A series of waves as experienced with 20th century pandemics, may lead to depletion of stocks of consumables, such as personal protective equipment and pharmaceuticals, before a second wave.
- Countries are encouraged to further estimate excess workplace absenteeism during a pandemic based on their own context and to guide all sectors to develop business continuity plans for high and possibly fluctuating levels of absenteeism throughout the pandemic.

Scientific basis

- Early reports and later analysis of epidemiological evidence suggest that milder epidemic waves (in Europe in April and May, 1918 and in the US in the spring of 1918) preceded the most severe pandemic wave in autumn 1918 (Frost WH, 1919; Olson SR et al., 2005).
- An influenza virus A(H1N1) resistant to oseltamivir was first reported from Norway in January 2008 and then spread throughout much of the Northern Hemisphere during the next couple of months (WHO, 2008). It subsequently was detected in the Southern Hemisphere during the summer of 2008.
- Excess mortality data from 1918 - 20 show that population mortality varied more than 30-fold across countries (Murray CL et al., 2006).
  - Variation among countries ranged from a low of 0.20% (Denmark) to a high of 4.39% (India).
  - Variation within countries ranged from 2.12% to 7.82% in India and from 0.25% to 1.00% in US.
- In the US during the 1918 pandemic, there were marked and consistent differences in

morbidity and to mortality among persons of different economic status: the lower the economic level, the higher the attack rate. This relationship persisted even after adjustments were made for factors such as colour, sex, age, and other conditions (Sydenstricker E, 1931).

- A multinational analysis of the 1968 pandemic showed very different epidemic patterns in the six countries studied (Viboud C et al., 2005).
  - In the US, a large epidemic was observed in 1968/1969, followed by a milder one in 1969/1970, late in the winter season.
  - In Canada, the two epidemic patterns were similar in amplitude and timing.
  - In other countries (Australia, France, the UK, and Japan), the first epidemic was mild, followed by a much more intense epidemic in the next season.
- A simulation study in the UK estimated that, overall, about 16% of the workforce is likely to be absent due to school closures during a pandemic. This estimate rises for sectors with a high proportion of female employees, such as health and social care (Sadique MZ et al., 2008).

Selected References

- Cockburn WC, Delon PJ, Ferreira W. **Origin and progress of the 1968-69 Hong Kong influenza epidemic.** Bull World Health Organ 1969;41:345-8.
- Murray CL, Lopez AD, Chin B et al. **Estimation of potential global pandemic influenza mortality on the basis of vital registry data from the 1918-20 pandemic: a quantitative analysis.** Lancet 2006;368:2211-18.
- Olson DR, Simonson L, Edelson PJ et al. **Epidemiological evidence of an early wave of the 1918 influenza pandemic in New York City.** PNAS 2005;102(31):11059-11063.
- Sadique MZ, Adams EJ, Edmunds WJ. **Estimating the costs of school closure for mitigating an influenza pandemic.** Public Health 2008, 8:135.
- Sydenstricker E. **The incidence of influenza among persons of different economic status during the epidemic of 1918.** Pub Health Report 1931;46(4) (republished in Pub Health Report, 2006;121(S1):191-204).
- Viboud C, Grais RF, Lafont BAP et al. **Multinational impact of the 1968 Hong Kong influenza pandemic: evidence for a smoldering pandemic.** JID 2005;192:233-48.
- WHO Expert committee on respiratory virus diseases. **First Report.** World Health Organization Technical Report Series No 170. Geneva, 1959.
- WHO. **Influenza A** (H1N1) **virus resistance to Oseltamivir :Preliminary summary and future plans.** WHO, Geneva, 2008 (at http://www.who.int/csr/disease/influenza/oseltamivir_ summary/en/index.html, accessed on 3 December 2008).

ANNEX 2 - REVISION PROCESS

On 27-29 November 2007, WHO convened the first meeting of the Pandemic Preparedness and Response Guidance Revision Working Group in Geneva, Switzerland. Experts in the field of communicable diseases and influenza, emergency and pandemic planning, and communications from national and international technical institutions, UN/international organizations and WHO staff from headquarters, regional and country offices convened to identify areas requiring updating.

The working group created five task forces with specific focus on developing a strategic policy document as well as recommendations on public health interventions, medical interventions, the "whole-of-society" approach to pandemic preparedness and communications.

In advance of an actual pandemic, the precise symptoms, epidemiology, virology and disease-transmission patterns can not be known. Assumptions based on past epidemics and seasonal influenza can, however, be used in order to facilitate pandemic preparedness planning activities - and identify disease control approaches likely to be effective. The assumptions upon which this guidance is based, outlined in Annex 1, were derived from available PubMed, Cochrane Library and secondary papers identified from existing relevant guidelines.

A second meeting of the Working Group was held on 05-07 March 2008 in Lyon, France. In order to support the discussions of Public Health Interventions and Medical Interventions Task Forces, WHO also hosted consultations in Geneva, Switzerland:

A final WHO consultation was convened on 05-09 May 2008 in Geneva, Switzerland to consolidate the results of these meetings to produce a draft of the strategic document.

The revised draft of the WHO Pandemic Preparedness Guidelines was made available for public review through the WHO web-site for four weeks. Over 600 comments from Member States, health related organizations, universities, the private sector and individuals were received. All input from this review were considered and evaluated by members of the task forces and the WHO Secretariat.

Declaration of Interest

WHO standard Declaration of Interest forms were completed by working group members as well as participants invited to WHO consultations, and reviewed by the WHO secretariat.

No conflicts of interest were declared among chairs and focal points of the five working group taskforces.

Three working group members reported their some conflicts of interest but none were considered as significant to proceed with the guideline revision process. The details are available upon request. Two other participants invited to three consultations reported some conflicts of interest but none were considered as significant to proceed with the guideline revision process.

Representatives from pharmaceutical industrial association were allowed to be present at a consultation on 05-09 May 2008 as observers.

Commenting process

The guidance was made available for public comments from 15 October to 3 November 2008. A message was posted to the WHO website indicating that anyone wishing to comment on the guidance contact the Global Influenza Programme. Those who wished to comment were provided with an electronic copy of the draft guidance and a Declaration of Interests Form. Following receipt of the Declaration of Interests Form and its approval, responders were provided with an account to access an electronic system to enter their comments. Many individuals and member states responded asking for more time to comment and the response period was extended to 10 November, and again to 15 November to accommodate two WHO Member States who requested a further extension.

428 individuals from 66 countries requested to review the guidance and provided 488 comments in the electronic forum. Over 150 written comments were also received from WHO Member States and other institutions via e-mail. These comments were analysed for duplication, categorized and resolved when possible (in the event of non-health related comments such a grammar or spelling). The remaining comments were reviewed in a series of four meetings with representative members of the working group and members of the WHO Secretariat on November 10, 17, 19 and 21. During these meetings, the comments were examined against the guidance and the relevant interventions analysed for effectiveness and feasibility. None of the comments processed during these meetings requested for a significant change in recommendations. Over 300 comments were accepted and integrated into the guidance, while approximately 200 comments were rejected in part or entirely. Reasons for rejection included the suggestion being a political commentary, an intervention determined as not sufficiently effective compared to cost, or a major conflict of interest on the part of the commenter (e.g. members of the pharmaceutical industry).

OVERVIEW OF STEPS FOR THE DEVELOPMENT OF PANDEMIC INFLUENZA PREPAREDNESS AND RESPONSE GUIDANCE REVISION

STEPS	DATE, PLACE	OUTCOME
1st Working Group Meeting	November 2007, Geneva	5 Task Forces to focus on various aspects of the guideline.
Drafting (EZ Collab discussions)	Nov.'07-Mar.'08, virtual space	1st draft of the guidelines.
1st Disease Control Strategies Task Force Meeting	January 2008, Geneva	2nd draft: Revised section on disease control strategies.
2nd Working Group Meeting	March 2008, Lyon	3rd draft of the guidelines.
Pandemic Surveillance Task Force Meeting	March 2008, Geneva	4th draft: Revised section on pandemic surveillance.
2nd Disease Control Strategies Task Force Meeting	April 2008, Geneva	5th draft: Revised section on disease control strategies.
Drafting (EZ Collab discussions)	Jan-May 2008, virtual space	6th draft: Collation of various sections.
Global Consultation for WHO Pandemic Preparedness Guidelines	May 2008, Geneva	7th draft: General consensus reached on main recommendations.
Revision, editing, visual elements	May-Oct 2008	8th draft.
Web based public review	Oct-Nov 2008	Over 600 comments received.
Processing of web based review comments	Dec. '08 - Jan '09	9th draft: comments incorporated into the document.
Internal WHO Clearance	February - April 2009	Official document ready for publication.